Bipolar Disorder Assessment and Treatment

Second Edition

Trisha Suppes, MD, PhD
Bipolar Disorder Research Program
VA Palo Alto Health Care System
Department of Psychiatry and Behavioral Sciences
Stanford University School of Medicine
Palo Alto, California

Ellen B. Dennehy, PhD
Department of Psychological Sciences
Purdue University
West Lafayette, Indiana
and
Bipolar Disorder Research Program
VA Palo Alto Health Care System
Palo Alto, California

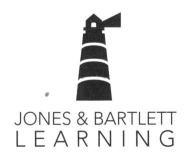

D1599880

JONES & BARTLETT
LEARNING

World Headquarters

Jones & Bartlett Learning
40 Tall Pine Drive
Sudbury, MA 01776
978-443-5000
info@jblearning.com
www.jblearning.com

Jones & Bartlett Learning Canada
6339 Ormindale Way
Mississauga, Ontario L5V 1J2
Canada

Jones & Bartlett Learning International
Barb House, Barb Mews
London W6 7PA
United Kingdom

Jones & Bartlett Learning books and products are available through most bookstores and online booksellers. To contact Jones & Bartlett Learning directly, call 800-832-0034, fax 978-443-8000, or visit our website, www.jblearning.com.

Substantial discounts on bulk quantities of Jones & Bartlett Learning publications are available to corporations, professional associations, and other qualified organizations. For details and specific discount information, contact the special sales department at Jones & Bartlett Learning via the above contact information or send an email to specialsales@jblearning.com.

The authors, editor, and publisher have made every effort to provide accurate information. However, they are not responsible for errors, omissions, or for any outcomes related to the use of the contents of this book and take no responsibility for the use of the products and procedures described. Treatments and side effects described in this book may not be applicable to all people; likewise, some people may require a dose or experience a side effect that is not described herein. Drugs and medical devices are discussed that may have limited availability controlled by the Food and Drug Administration (FDA) for use only in a research study or clinical trial. Research, clinical practice, and government regulations often change the accepted standard in this field. When consideration is being given to use of any drug in the clinical setting, the healthcare provider or reader is responsible for determining FDA status of the drug, reading the package insert, and reviewing prescribing information for the most up-to-date recommendations on dose, precautions, and contraindications, and determining the appropriate usage for the product. This is especially important in the case of drugs that are new or seldom used.

Production Credits

Executive Publisher: Christopher Davis
Editorial Assistant: Sara Cameron
Production Editor: Daniel Stone
Production Director: Amy Rose
Associate Marketing Manager: Katie Hennessy
V.P., Manufacturing and Inventory Control: Therese Connell
Project Management: Thistle Hill Publishing Services, LLC
Composition: Dedicated Business Solutions, Inc.
Cover Design: Kristin E. Parker
Cover Image: © Robert O. Brown Photography/ ShutterStock, Inc.
Printing and Binding: Malloy, Incorporated
Cover Printing: Malloy, Incorporated

Library of Congress Cataloging-in-Publication Data

Bipolar disorder assessment and treatment / Trisha Suppes, Ellen B. Dennehy. — 2nd ed.
  p. ; cm.
  Rev. ed. of: Bipolar disorder : treatment and management / by Trisha Suppes, Paul E. Keck Jr. c2005.
  Includes bibliographical references and index.
  ISBN-13: 978-0-7637-9765-2 (pbk.)
  ISBN-10: 0-7637-9765-0 (pbk.)
  1. Manic-depressive illness. 2. Manic-depressive illness—Treatment. I. Dennehy, Ellen B., 1968- II. Suppes, Trisha. Bipolar disorder. III. Title.
  [DNLM: 1. Bipolar Disorder—diagnosis. 2. Bipolar Disorder—therapy. WM 207]
  RC516.S865 2012
  616.89'5—dc22
                2010040260

6048

Printed in the United States of America
14 13 12 11 10 10 9 8 7 6 5 4 3 2 1

Contents

Chapter 1: General Information about Bipolar Disorder   1

What Is Bipolar Disorder? 1

What Is the Role of Genetics in Bipolar Disorder?. 4

How Does Brain Anatomy and Physiology Differ for Patients with Bipolar
   Disorder?. 5

    Specific Brain Areas Involved in Bipolar Disorder 5

    Biochemical and Physiological Factors Related to Bipolar Disorder 7

    Secondary Messenger Systems 7

How Does the Disorder Affect Patients' Lives?. 8

    Specific Impact of Mania 8

    Specific Impact of Hypomania 9

    Specific Impact of Depression 9

    Specific Impact of Mixed Episodes 10

How Common Is Bipolar Disorder?. 11

What Is the Likelihood of Recovery? 11

Chapter 2: Diagnosing and Assessing Bipolar Disorder   13

What Are the Typical Symptoms of Bipolar Disorder?. 13

    Recognizing Symptoms of Mania 14

    Recognizing Symptoms of Hypomania 15

    Recognizing Symptoms of Depression 16

    Recognizing a Mixed Episode 16

What Are the Criteria for Diagnosing Bipolar Disorder? 17

    Diagnostic Specifiers for Bipolar I Disorder and Bipolar II Disorder 17

    Course Specifiers 19

What Tools Exist for Diagnosing Bipolar Disorder? 19

    Conducting a Medical Assessment. 20

    Conducting the Clinical Interview 21

    Using Structured Symptom Evaluation Tools 21

    Assessing Suicide Risk 25

What Differentiates Bipolar Disorder from Other Disorders? 26

How Does Bipolar Disorder Present in Children and Adolescents? 29

Chapter 3: Biological Treatment of Bipolar Disorder   31

What Medications Have Received Approval from the Food and Drug Administration for Treatment of Bipolar Disorders? 32

What Are Treatment Guidelines for Bipolar Disorder? 33

What Medications Are Used to Treat Mania/Hypomania in Patients with Bipolar Disorder? 33

    Effectiveness of Medications for Treating Mania/Hypomania Symptoms of Bipolar Disorder 38

    Using Combination Medications 41

What Medications Are Used to Treat Depression in Patients with Bipolar Disorder? 42

    Effectiveness of Medications for Treating Depression in Bipolar Disorder 45

What Strategies Are Recommended for Maintenance Treatment? 48

    Effectiveness of Maintenance Treatment for Bipolar Patients 48

How Can Medication Treatment of Side Effects Be Managed? 51

How Are Electroconvulsive Therapy (ECT) and Alternative Medicine Used to Treat Patients with Bipolar Disorder? 51

How Does the Presence of Co-Occurring Disorders Impact Medication Treatment for Bipolar Disorder? 53

Chapter 4: Psychosocial Treatments for Bipolar Disorder   55

Why Add Psychosocial Interventions to Pharmacotherapy? 55

    Improving Adherence to Medication Treatment 56

    Coping with Stress 57

    Preventing Relapse 58

    Improving Functioning and Quality of Life 58

What Psychosocial Interventions Are Used to Treat Bipolar Disorder? 59

What Is the Psychoeducational Approach to Bipolar Disorder Treatment? 61

    Psychoeducational Treatment Strategies 61

    Effectiveness of Psychoeducation 63

What Is Family-Focused Treatment (FFT) for Bipolar Disorder? 64

    FFT Treatment Strategies 64

    Effectiveness of FFT 65

What Individual Psychosocial Therapy Approaches Are Used to Treat Bipolar Disorder? 67

    CBT Treatment Strategies 67

    Effectiveness of CBT 69

IPSRT Strategies. 70

Effectiveness of IPSRT. 72

Which Psychosocial Approaches Are Best for the Treatment of Bipolar Disorder?. **73**

Comparisons of Different Therapeutic Approaches 73

Appendix A: *DSM-IV–TR* **Diagnostic Criteria.** **77**

Appendix B: Tools for Diagnosis and Assessment of Bipolar Disorder. **87**

Appendix C: Life Chart Sample. **95**

Glossary. **99**

References. **103**

Index **119**

Chapter 1
General Information about Bipolar Disorder

This chapter answers the following questions:

▶ **What Is Bipolar Disorder?**—This section defines the disorder, introduces possible causes, and presents the four categories of diagnoses associated with the disorder.

▶ **What Is the Role of Genetics in Bipolar Disorder?**—This section reviews research on the genetic inheritance of bipolar disorder.

▶ **How Do Brain Anatomy and Physiology Differ for Patients with Bipolar Disorder?**—This section covers how neuroimaging studies have helped define the areas of the brain involved in bipolar disorder.

▶ **How Does the Disorder Affect Patients' Lives?**—This section covers the impact of mania, hypomania, depression, and mixed episodes on patients' lives.

▶ **How Common Is Bipolar Disorder?**—This section gives prevalence rates for the United States and Europe.

▶ **What Is the Likelihood of Recovery?**—This section discusses the importance of treatment plan compliance in reducing symptoms of the disorder.

OR those with bipolar disorder, as well as for their families and friends, life is an unpredictable and debilitating series of emotional highs and lows. Referred to in the past as manic-depression, bipolar disorder represents a biological condition characterized by rapid mood swings. A manic episode brings on euphoria, recklessness, compromised financial security, and relationship problems. When the pendulum swings to a depressive episode, there is extreme hopelessness and listlessness.

Originally, mania was a nonspecific term for madness, and melancholia was a type of "madness" characterized by a withdrawn and quiet demeanor.

Today, more than 5.7 million American adults suffer from bipolar disorder (Kessler et al., 2005a). The first episodes typically appear in adolescence or early adulthood when life stresses are at their greatest. For women, bipolar disorder may be triggered by childbirth or menopause.

Although there is no single, documented cause or known cure for bipolar disorder, medications and other therapies can help manage the symptoms. Without treatment, the course of illness can worsen, with episodes becoming more frequent, intense, and characterized by more psychotic behavior.

What Is Bipolar Disorder?

"Mania" and "melancholia"—ancient terms for two distinct mood changes—characterize the disorder today referred to as bipolar disorder. Historically, 19th-century physicians

mania—a mood state characterized by an elevated or irritable mood, decreased sleep, high energy or activity, impulsive behavior, and increased goal-directed behavior

depression—a mood state characterized by sadness or irritability, low energy, thoughts of death and suicide, and lack of interest in previously enjoyed activities

impulsivity—taking action with limited thought to consequences

hypomania—a mood state characterized by increased energy, excitement, and changes in mood that do not meet the diagnostic criteria for a full manic episode

PET imaging—technology that uses positron-labeled molecules and an oxygen blood flow tracer to develop images of brain activity versus the structural images provided by MRI

euthymia—normal range of mood, no evidence of mania, hypomania, or depression

Chapters 3 and 4 detail appropriate treatment choices for varied symptom patterns.

recognized alternating episodes of *mania* and *depression* as distinct disorders, and, by the early 1900s, bipolar disorder was distinguished from schizophrenia. In 1952, the first edition of the *Diagnostic and Statistical Manual of Mental Disorders* presented an early conceptualization of the disorder (American Psychiatric Association [APA], 1952).

Bipolar disorder is a mood disorder characterized by significant swings between mania and depression, as well as changes in sleep patterns, energy, activity, attention, and *impulsivity*. Although there are many variations of mood patterns and severity that a person with bipolar disorder might experience, he or she generally experiences periods of mood elevation (mania and/or *hypomania*) and major depressive episodes. Some of these episodes are "mixed," meaning that symptoms of both mania and depression are present during the same episode. Patients may also experience psychotic symptoms when manic or depressed.

Although the exact cause of bipolar disorder is unknown, both genetic and environmental factors may contribute to its development and course. Possible environmental factors include substance abuse, medical problems (e.g., thyroid fluctuation), stressful life events, and lifestyles that interfere with routine sleep-wake cycles. Through *PET imaging*, which detects differences in the brain activity of people who are depressed or manic compared to those experiencing a normal mood state, as well as other biological research, researchers are gaining a better understanding of the causes of bipolar disorder. As a result, experts now believe that a dysregulation (not unlike an epileptic seizure) occurs in the brain cells regulating emotions, circadian rhythms, and behaviors, thus causing bipolar symptoms (Goodwin & Jamison, 2007).

One challenging feature of bipolar disorder is that patients' experience of the illness can vary tremendously, with some patients suffering depression followed by hypomania, and others mania followed by depression. Some move quickly from episode to episode, with virtually no period of mood stability (*euthymia*) between significant ups and downs. Others may be relatively stable between discrete episodes of mania or depression for longer periods. Defining an individual's characteristic pattern is important and can affect choice of treatments.

The graph in Figure 1.1 illustrates these varying patterns in two patients: Sue, a 55-year-old secretary and John, a 28-year-old unemployed construction worker.

Epidemiological studies suggest that the average age of onset for first episode is 18.2 years for those with bipolar I disorder, and 20.3 years for those with bipolar II disorder (Merikangas

Figure 1.1 Individual Characteristic Patterns

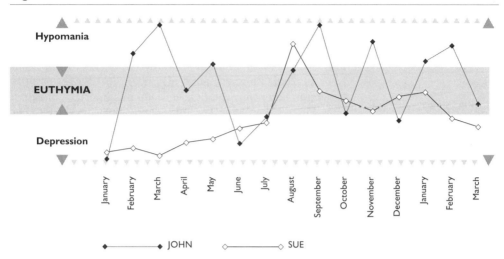

et al., 2007). A person's first significant episode is often associated with stressful life events, such as beginning a new job, going to college, getting married, or having a child. Importantly, the average time from symptom onset to correct diagnosis may be eight to nine years. This is likely at least in part due to the difficulty in recognizing the gradual development of bipolar symptoms (Schaffer, Cairney, Cheung, Veldhuizen, & Levitt, 2006; Wang et al., 2005).

Over time, the duration of "well" periods between mood episodes can decrease in some individuals, leading to a more chronic, severe course with more episodes of mania or depression. Others may start out experiencing one episode per year and continue at this frequency. Studies conducted in the early 1900s (before medication treatment) indicate that some patients experienced less time between episodes as they aged. For example, in the early days of their illness, the characteristic course for one individual might have been three to four years between episodes; however, as they aged, they might have experienced 12–18 months between mood episodes. This is still the course of the illness for some patients, who have a range of presentations and course of illness patterns. However, others develop chronic ongoing symptoms, with few days of relatively symptom-free functioning between acute episodes. Evidence suggests that those who experience more episodes before treatment begins may develop greater resistance to treatment, making early detection and intervention important (Swann et al., 1997).

An area of continued research and debate revolves around the possibility of broadening bipolar disorder diagnostic criteria to include a spectrum of mood manifestations not meeting current *DSM–IV* criteria for a bipolar diagnosis. For example, some see "bipolarity" as a dimensional illness that includes continuous mood symptoms from the most severe through entities not currently categorized by *DSM–IV–TR* (e.g., borderline bipolar, soft bipolar, and affective temperaments, such as hyperthymic, cyclothymic, dysthymic, irritable) (Angst et al., 2003; Benazzi, 2007; Zimmerman et al., 2009). Further research is needed to determine the link between this interface of symptoms and "temperament" and subsequent implications for illness course and treatment.

In recent decades, we have come to understand that bipolar disorder typically stems from instability and malfunction in brain activity, not from environmental causes. However, we continue to have a limited and rudimentary understanding of the exact mechanisms underlying the disorder. The field is advancing at a rapid rate as findings in brain research and the neurosciences expand.

During depression, the frontal cortex will show decreased activation; during mania, temporal lobe regions will show increased activation. Researchers believe that changes in activation can be correlated with blood flow and brain activity.

What Is the Role of Genetics in Bipolar Disorder?

Bipolar disorder is now recognized as an inherited illness likely caused by interactions of multiple genes (Faraone, Glatt, & Tsuang, 2003; Hayden & Nurnberger, 2006; Smoller & Finn, 2003).

When assessing individuals with possible bipolar disorder, it is important to ask about history of bipolar disorder, depression, substance abuse, and suicide in their family members.

Several respected European adoption studies have found the possibility of developing bipolar disorder to be higher for children who had a birth parent diagnosed with bipolar disorder,

From the Patient's Perspective

The doctor says there is a connection between all my energy right now and how depressed I was feeling last winter, and that I have something called "bipolar disorder." Now, I'm supposed to take "mood stabilizing" medication. I didn't think that these problems were that bad, and I am a little surprised that she thinks I need medicine. However, I've been on it for a few weeks now, and I do feel better. I am getting better sleep and feel more in control of myself. Hopefully, it will prevent me from getting depressed again, too. I am going to miss that extra energy, but she says that bipolar disorder is a biological illness, and I have to take it seriously and stick with treatment so it won't get worse.

whether or not the child was raised with that individual (Faraone & Tsuang, 2003; Smoller & Finn, 2003). In addition, twin studies indicate a much higher risk (50 percent) for identical twins than for fraternal twins (about 15–20 percent) (Goodwin & Jamison, 2007).

Among family members with bipolar disorder, the risk for other psychiatric illnesses is significantly elevated as well. For any given individual with bipolar disorder, the likelihood of family members having depression is significant, at least as much as bipolar disorder itself. The risk for other coexisting psychiatric illnesses is also high, including substance abuse and anxiety disorders. Members of families in which more than one person has bipolar disorder or depression can experience both earlier onset and a more severe course of bipolar disorder (McElroy et al., 2001; Suppes et al., 2001).

> When one parent has bipolar disorder, the risk to each child can be 15–20 percent. When both parents have bipolar disorder, the risk increases to 50–75 percent.

Stress management is an important treatment goal for persons with bipolar disorder, as stress can increase vulnerability to clinical symptoms and/or episodes. For example, sleep deprivation or significant psychosocial stress could predispose someone currently stable to experience a new episode. Some theorists also suggest that patients may carry the genetic predisposition to bipolar disorder, but do not develop symptoms unless exposed to significant stress, especially during developmental periods (Padmos et al., 2009). For example, extensive use of illegal substances or early physical or sexual trauma could trigger this stress vulnerability.

How Does Brain Anatomy and Physiology Differ for Patients with Bipolar Disorder?

This section addresses specific brain areas involved in the disorder as well as relevant biochemical and physiological factors and secondary messenger systems within nerve cells.

Specific Brain Areas Involved in Bipolar Disorder

Brain areas involved when people are depressed and manic include the frontal lobe (where the brain performs many of its *executive* and organizational functions) and temporal lobes (involved in regulating emotions). For years, theorists implicated the *temporal lobe*, which includes the *hippocampus* and the *amygdala*, in the development of affective instability, including depression, bipolar disorder, and aggression. For example, those with epilepsy syndromes localized to the temporal lobe (specifically, the hippocampus) develop many bipolar-like symptoms, including

executive functions—those functions of the brain carried out by the prefrontal and frontal cortex: managing stimuli, marshalling appropriate responses, and modulating impulses, which are all disrupted in the manic state

temporal lobe—a large lobe of each cerebral hemisphere that is in front of the occipital lobe and is believed to be involved in memory, mood regulation, and impulsivity

hippocampus—an important part of the limbic system involved in working memory and other functions

amygdala—one of the basal ganglia that is part of the limbic system and believed to be involved in impulsivity and other functions

Figure 1.2   Brain Areas Impacted by Bipolar Disorder

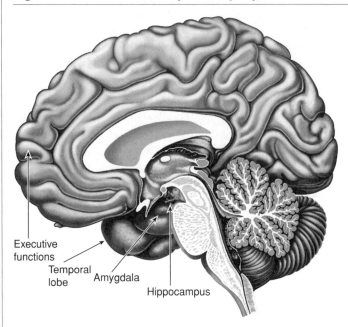

Executive functions

Temporal lobe   Amygdala

Hippocampus

paranormal phenomena—altered perceptions experienced by the patient but not those around him or her (e.g., auditory hallucinations [hearing voices, for example], olfactory hallucinations [smelling burning rubber], and also déjà vu [the sense of having already experienced what is now happening])

SPECT imaging—a single photon emission where image intensity is directly correlated to cerebral perfusion or blood flow, which is believed to be related to brain functional activity

We cannot use neuroimaging technologies to diagnose a specific illness or to predict the most effective treatment approach.

unstable moods and *paranormal phenomena*. Figure 1.2 illustrates the specific brain areas impacted by bipolar disorder.

With current neuroimaging technology—PET and *SPECT imaging*—we can now:

▶ Identify some brain areas involved in the disorder.

▶ Establish that the brain is physiologically different, depending on the mood state the person is experiencing.

▶ Assess differences in patients' brains when they experience depression versus mania versus euthymia (see Figure 1.3 for an example).

▶ Demonstrate how brain function normalizes after medication treatment, indicating that medications effectively return brain activity to more balanced function.

Figure 1.3   Brain Function by SPECT Imaging Scan

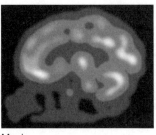

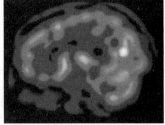

Mania   No clinical evidence of mania

Biochemical and Physiological Factors Related to Bipolar Disorder

Much of the biochemical theory about bipolar disorder stems from our understanding of drug mechanisms, expanding as novel medications have been found effective in the treatment of this illness. Nineteenth-century thinking was that mental illnesses and bipolar disorder were due to the deposit of salt on the brain tissue itself. As a result, by the mid-1800s, lithium bromide was recommended by physicians to treat mania and melancholia as both an acute and prophylactic treatment. Despite advances in our understanding of the physiologic basis of brain activity, this potentially effective treatment was lost until the 1950s (Cade, 1949). While earlier schools of thought debated what caused bipolar disorder—whether the *neurotransmitter*, norepinephrine, regulated moods or *dopamine* was related to psychoses—researchers now understand that interactions producing both abnormal brain states and relative stability are much more complex than originally thought. For example, in evaluating how *second-generation antipsychotics* impact the brain's *major neurochemical receptor group*, debate continues as to whether more *serotonin* versus less serotonin, more dopamine versus less dopamine (or the combination of the two) are the critical components of mood stabilization.

Secondary Messenger Systems

Historically, psychiatric research focused on receptor activity (i.e., the activity at the cell surface). Now, many studies are ongoing to better understand the specific mechanisms inside the neuronal cell associated with symptoms of bipolar disorder and how medications to treat bipolar disorder act on the brain. Studies in patients treated with lithium and other compounds (especially anticonvulsant medications) suggest a disruption (e.g., too much or too little of a second messenger molecule) and that treatment corrects this imbalance, leading to mood stabilization.

This focus on second messengers has also led to an awareness of a potential *neuroprotective effect* of many anti-manic medications. Lithium and many of the anticonvulsants appear to have a protective effect in animal models where there is a decreased loss of already existing cells and evidence showing an increased likelihood of new neurogenesis (Manji, Moore, & Chen, 2000).

New areas of research are also focusing on brain effects of:

▶ **Neuropeptides**—Brain chemicals or medications that either decrease cell death and/or increase neurogenesis.

---

neurotransmitter—a chemical in the brain that transmits information between the nerve cells

dopamine—a neurotransmitter in the central nervous system that affects the synthesis of epinephrine

second-generation antipsychotics—the class of antipsychotic medications with fewer extrapyramidal side effects; although the medications in this class share this benefit, they have very different mechanisms of action

major neurochemical receptor groups—neurotransmitter substances believed important in normal and abnormal brain functioning

serotonin—a neurotransmitter from the indoleamine group that affects central nervous system functioning

neuroprotective effect—the function of a brain chemical or medication to either decrease cell death and/or increase the birth of new brain cells (i.e., neurogenesis)

Research in recent years has turned to the next level of brain function—secondary messenger systems— neurochemical systems used to carry and communicate activity from a cell's surface throughout the cell body and into the areas that determine the cell's genetic products.

▶ **Cotransmitters**—Two molecules released from the same synapse that act on an adjacent neuron, both of which are physiologically active.

▶ **Hormone receptors** (e.g., steroid receptors)—A group of molecules that have diverse function throughout the brain and the body (e.g., estrogen).

▶ **Neurotrophins**—A class of molecules whose effects occur through specific cell membrane receptors that trigger changes in the second messenger system(s). These effects range from increased cell survival to increased new cell growth.

As a result, we can expect important new findings in the next 10 years on fundamental brain processes and underlying mechanisms of major psychiatric illnesses.

How Does the Disorder Affect Patients' Lives?

Those with bipolar disorder typically find that their quality of life and ability to function changes, even with adequate treatment and symptom remission (Coryell et al., 1993; Judd et al., 2005; Tohen et al., 2000).

Specific Impact of Mania

circadian rhythms—the daily regulation of sleep-wake cycles and activity-to-activity patterns

Typically, those experiencing a manic episode find they sleep less or not at all due to a disruption in their *circadian rhythms*. Despite this, they sustain high energy levels (e.g., a person in a full manic episode may feel little or no need for sleep, exercise several hours daily, and have "boundless" energy for new projects). This increase in energy may be observed as an increase in activity. However, it may not be focused in a productive fashion, and the patient may go for many days without sleeping. In fact, patients in the 19th century (prior to medication treatment) would sometimes die from manic episodes due to lack of sleep and neglecting to eat or drink water.

grandiosity—exaggerated belief or claims of one's importance or identity; manifested as delusions of great wealth, power, or fame when of psychotic proportions

Classic mania is also associated with *grandiosity* and behavior that family and friends recognize as atypical for the individual, such as spending sprees, promiscuity, alcohol or drug abuse, or other impulsive, potentially risky behavior. Patients with bipolar disorder may neither recognize their symptoms nor, as mania worsens, the consequences of their risky behavior because of the loss of contact with reality that occurs when the disorder remains untreated. Mania can profoundly disrupt an individual's life, often leading to joblessness, financial instability, and damaged family relationships.

The Impact of Bipolar Disorder and Substance Abuse

In general, impact of bipolar disorder may be more serious when associated with other disorders, such as alcohol and drug abuse (Frye et al., 2003; McElroy et al., 2001). Compared to the general population, men and women with bipolar disorder are four times and eight times, respectively, more likely to become alcoholic (Regier et al., 1990).

Substance abuse may have a cumulative impact on the brain, affecting course and treatment response. For example, one study found that a history of substance abuse further complicates the course of bipolar disorder and has significant treatment implications, such as lower rates of remission and poor response to lithium (Goldberg, Carno, Leon, Kocsis, & Portera, 1999). In addition, substance use is associated with poor treatment compliance (Perlick, 2004; Strakowski, DelBello, Fleck, & Arndt, 2000). Thus, patients must be cautioned against substance abuse, and use of substances needs to be discussed routinely in clinical visits.

More than 50 percent of those with bipolar disorder will experience a lifetime prevalence of alcohol and/or substance abuse or dependence.

Specific Impact of Hypomania

Those experiencing hypomania feel "on top of the world," able to accomplish more than usual, sociable, creative, and invigorated. Thus, these symptoms are rarely reported as problems or concerns as patients perceive them to be positive and beneficial. For those with bipolar I disorder, untreated hypomania typically progresses to mania. While the experience of hypomania is not as severe as mania, hypomania also increases the likelihood of making impulsive decisions, which can have lasting negative consequences, and persons in a hypomanic episode experience a change from usual functioning that is noticeable by others. Many episodes of hypomania are "mixed," in which patients experience some depressive symptoms within a hypomanic episode. Recent work suggests that as many as 57 percent of hypomanic episodes are mixed, and that this is more common for women (Suppes et al., 2005).

Specific Impact of Depression

Depression often impacts people's sleeping and eating habits, causing some to:

- ▶ Wake up feeling tired from being up and down all night and waking earlier than usual.
- ▶ Sleep far more than normal.
- ▶ Have little or no appetite.
- ▶ Gain weight from overeating.
- ▶ Find food unsatisfying or unappealing.

Depressed people often have trouble concentrating, remembering, and making decisions. They may be unable to concentrate on a television program or book, decide what to wear, or decide

Suicides, suicide attempts, and suicidal ideation are more likely to occur when patients are experiencing either depressed or mixed episodes (APA, 2000). Chapter 2 includes a section on assessing suicide risk (pp. 25–26).

whether to renew a subscription, feeling that these decisions are overwhelming or exhausting. Persons with depression report very low self-esteem and often dwell on their negative qualities, failings, or losses. They also report feelings of hopelessness: a belief that nothing will ever improve, and exaggerated pessimism.

Specific Impact of Mixed Episodes

Many patients experience a mix of symptoms, with depressive symptoms either occurring simultaneously or within a short time of hypomanic or manic symptoms. For example, a patient could be very irritable and depressed but also feel restless, with an excess of energy or activation. When patients meet criteria for a full depressive episode and a full manic episode at the same time, it is called a "mixed episode."

Patients may also experience mixed symptoms without meeting full criteria for both mania and depression. This expression of mixed symptoms is not recognized as a mixed "episode" in the current classifications of bipolar disorder allowed in the *DSM–IV–TR*, but it is a common expression of symptoms in those with bipolar disorders. For example, a patient may be in a hypomanic episode but have significant depressive symptoms as well. Clinicians may think of these patterns as *mixed hypomania* or "mixed depression," depending on whether depressive or hypomanic symptoms are predominant.

mixed hypomania—this term describes those individuals who meet the criteria for hypomania but also experience simultaneous symptoms of dysphoria and depression that do not meet the full criteria for a depressive episode

Bipolar disorder may also be accompanied by a high risk for self-injury and suicide when symptoms persist untreated, patients fail to take medications as prescribed or are actively abusing substances, or when patients experience a limited response to treatment (Baldessarini & Tondo, 2008; Tondo, Isacsson, & Baldessarini, 2003).

From the Patient's Perspective

I can't believe how productive I am! Like today . . . It's 2:15 a.m., and I am still going strong. Just finished buying some new Christmas decorations online, started cleaning the house, fixed the kids' lunches for the week. Next, I'm going to tackle the office paperwork. I even worked out! I hope this extra energy lasts; I don't know what I did to deserve this, but I feel great. I feel very competent, happy, and productive; it sure feels better than the "down-in-the-dumps" winter I had.

How Common Is Bipolar Disorder?

The latest estimates of bipolar disorder prevalence in the United States indicate that about 2 percent of people meet criteria for either bipolar I or bipolar II disorder (Kessler et al., 2005b; Merikangas et al., 2007). When the definitions for the illness are broadened slightly, as is often advocated, these numbers increase to about 5 percent of the population (Merikangas et al., 2007). Importantly, about 30 percent of people with the illness have either been diagnosed and are not receiving treatment, are undiagnosed, or have been diagnosed in error—usually as having major depressive disorder alone.

What Is the Likelihood of Recovery?

Bipolar disorder is a lifelong, recurrent illness. Once it is diagnosed, continued consultation and treatment is necessary to reduce symptoms and maintain remission. Treatment commonly involves taking one or more medications. Patients can improve their prognosis by:

► Cooperating with health care professionals and their treatment plan

► Taking medications as directed

► Detecting changes in symptoms early by monitoring their moods and behaviors

► Enhancing their brain chemistry by making healthy diet and exercise choices

Sudden discontinuation of prescribed medications can worsen bipolar disorder by reducing the patient's response to medication in the future and/or increasing the frequency of episodes.

Those with untreated bipolar disorder are typically unstable, experiencing uncomfortable and unpredictable mood states as well as changes in energy, sleep, and behavior. Even when treated, medications may have to be adjusted as patients face new episodes or breakthrough symptoms. However, with effective medication treatment, many patients experience a significant reduction or remission in symptoms.

This book is intended for health care professionals, but may also be helpful to consumers and family members. Clinicians working with patients with bipolar disorder will find information to supplement their work, as follows:

► **Chapter 2** covers assessment and diagnostic techniques as well as how to differentiate between bipolar disorder and other disorders with similar symptoms.

► **Chapter 3** addresses pharmacological and other biologically based treatment approaches.

► **Chapter 4** covers psychosocial treatment approaches used in conjunction with medication therapy.

▶ **Appendix A** presents the *DSM–IV–TR* criteria for bipolar disorder.

▶ **Appendix B** includes detailed information on assessment tools listed in Chapter 2.

▶ **Appendix C** includes a sample log from the Life Chart, a self-report method for documenting bipolar symptoms.

Key Concepts for Chapter 1

1. Bipolar disorder is a medical-biological illness with a genetic component related to changes in brain activity.

2. Bipolar disorder is characterized by extremes in mood and energy that vary from one patient to another in duration, intensity, order of occurrence, and length of symptom-free period between episodes.

3. When symptoms persist untreated, medication compliance is low, or when there is limited response to treatment, patients with bipolar disorder may have a high risk for self-injury and suicide.

4. Patients often fail to recognize manic symptoms, especially if they become confused and lose contact with reality as mania worsens. Also, patients with hypomanic symptoms may fail to report these symptoms as they perceive them to be positive and beneficial.

5. There is a strong association between bipolar disorder and alcohol and/or substance abuse or dependence with a history of either signifying a potentially more severe course of illness and less response to treatment.

6. Bipolar disorder is a lifelong, recurrent illness that can be treated with medications and psychosocial interventions.

Chapter 2
Diagnosing and Assessing Bipolar Disorder

This chapter answers the following questions:

▶ **What Are the Typical Symptoms of Bipolar Disorder?**—This section reviews the typical symptoms of mania, hypomania, and depression.

▶ **What Are the Criteria for Diagnosing Bipolar Disorder?**—This section presents the *DSM–IV–TR* criteria for making a diagnosis as well as diagnostic clarifiers.

▶ **What Tools Exist for Diagnosing Bipolar Disorder?**—This section offers direction on conducting medical assessments and clinical interviews as well as using clinician- and self-rated assessment tools.

▶ **What Differentiates Bipolar Disorder from Other Disorders?**—This section reviews the various physiological and psychological disorders that may be difficult to distinguish from bipolar diagnoses or coexist with bipolar disorder.

▶ **How Does Bipolar Disorder Present in Children and Adolescents?**—This section gives an overview of issues related to diagnosing and treating bipolar disorder in these age groups.

ASSESSING bipolar disorder involves identifying the patient's range of episodes, including depression, mania or hypomania, and dysphoric or *mixed episodes*. Other factors that help specify the diagnosis include *rapid cycling* and whether *psychosis* is present during mood episodes.

Patients who present for treatment may not reveal all the dimensions of their mood fluctuations; thus, thorough assessment is critical to detect bipolar disorder. In particular, this may occur because of lack of insight, failure to recognize symptoms or to identify them as problematic, or a reluctance to take medications or to be labeled as having an "illness." For example, research demonstrates that many patients seek help while in a depressive episode and may not spontaneously volunteer information regarding past episodes of hypomania or mania, or even recognize them as problematic or part of the same illness pattern (Akiskal, 1996; Benazzi, 2000; Bowden, 2001). It is critical that clinicians ask specifically about these types of mood symptoms when first evaluating a depressed patient.

What Are the Typical Symptoms of Bipolar Disorder?

The symptoms of mania, hypomania, and depression are recognizable and relatively similar from patient to patient. Figure 2.1 provides an overview of manic, hypomanic, and depressive symptoms. What differs across patients is the amount of time

mixed episodes—periods during which criteria for both a manic and depressive episode are met during the same period of time.

rapid cycling—four or more manic, hypomanic, or depressive episodes in any 12-month period

psychosis—extreme impairment of a person's ability to think clearly, perceive things accurately, respond emotionally, communicate effectively, understand reality, and behave appropriately

"Dysphoria" derives from a Greek word meaning "distress" or "hard to bear" and is used by the psychiatric and medical community as a diagnostic term generally referring to subthreshold depression that does not meet the full criteria for a major depressive episode.

spent in each type of episode and frequency of episodes, the experience of persistent subsyndromal symptoms between significant mood episodes, and the amount of time spent "well."

Recognizing Symptoms of Mania

Manic symptoms can appear as the following:

> ► **A highly excited, energetic mood state**—Feeling "on top of the world" and able to achieve anything despite a decreased ability to complete necessary tasks. Those with mania feel they need very little sleep or rest. They may spend excessively, participate in indiscriminate social/sexual interactions, or act impulsively. Although the manic individual may feel happy and expansive, friends and family will recognize their behavior as excessive and may refer the person for treatment. Untreated, mania will worsen, with moods becoming more elevated or irritable, behavior more unpredictable, and judgment more impaired. These individuals are often unaware of the consequences of their extreme behavior due to lack of insight, altered judgment, disorientation, and loss of contact with reality.

Figure 2.1 provides an overview of manic, hypomanic, and depressive symptoms.

Figure 2.1   Overview of Manic, Hypomanic, and Depressive Symptoms

Symptoms of Mania	Symptoms of Hypomania	Symptoms of Depression
• Increased physical and mental activity/energy • Heightened mood, exaggerated optimism, and self-confidence • Excessive irritability, aggressive behavior • Decreased need for sleep without feeling fatigued • Ambitious or grandiose plans, inflated sense of self-importance • Increased or more rapid speech than normal • More thoughts than normal, racing thoughts, flight of ideas • Impulsiveness, poor judgment, distractibility • Reckless behavior • Increased sexual interest and/or activity • In severe cases, delusions and hallucinations	• Similar to manic symptoms, but not as severe and duration can be shorter • Increased physical and mental activity/energy • Heightened mood, exaggerated optimism, and self-confidence • Excessive irritability • Decreased need for sleep without feeling fatigued • More talkative than usual • More thoughts than normal, racing thoughts, flight of ideas • Distractibility • Increase in goal-directed activity or psychomotor agitation • Reckless behavior • Increased sexual interest and/or activity	• Prolonged sadness or unexplained crying spells • Significant changes in appetite and sleep patterns • Irritability, anger, worry, agitation, anxiety • Pessimism, indifference • Loss of energy, persistent lethargy • Feelings of guilt, worthlessness • Inability to concentrate, indecisiveness • Inability to take pleasure in former interests, social withdrawal • Unexplained aches and pains • Recurring thoughts of death or suicide

▶ **An irritable, excited mood**—Moods fluctuate between euphoria and irritability, all charged by excessive energy, restlessness, and agitation. Similar to classic mania, the patient will have a subjective sense of racing thoughts and, while initiating many projects, will finish few.

When manic, about 50 percent of patients experience symptoms of psychosis (including *delusions* and *hallucinations*), which may further impair judgment and contribute to erratic behavior.

A **manic episode** is defined by a distinct period of persistently elevated, expansive, or irritable mood **lasting at least one week** (or less if hospitalization is required). The mood is also accompanied by additional symptoms, such as those highlighted above.

Recognizing Symptoms of Hypomania

Hypomania resembles mania, but symptoms do not meet full criteria for a manic episode and are rarely reported for psychiatric intervention, as the person may perceive the experience as positive. Hypomanic individuals experience discrete periods of time when they feel on top of things, productive, sociable, and self-confident. They feel excited, energized, creative, active, intelligent, and sometimes more sexual. They may say that they feel better than at any other time in their lives and fail to recognize errors in judgment, neglect of everyday duties, or other subtle lapses in functioning. They cannot understand why anyone would call their experience abnormal or part of a disorder.

Although the preceding paragraph describes a pure hypomanic episode, many patients (particularly women) experience mixed symptoms when hypomanic, perhaps having increased irritability, anger, or sadness in conjunction with extra physical and mental energy (Suppes et al., 2005). For some individuals, mixed hypomania may be experienced as an "energized depression."

One of the criteria for diagnosing hypomania is a change of state **observable by others**. This noticeable change of state can be best verified by talking with family members or close associates who can comment on previous behavior.

A **hypomanic episode** is defined by a distinct period of persistently elevated, expansive, or irritable mood **lasting at least four days**. The mood is also accompanied by additional symptoms: inflated self-esteem or grandiosity, a decreased need for sleep, pressured speech, flight of ideas, distractibility, increased involvement in goal-directed activities or psychomotor agitation, and excessive involvement in pleasurable and high-risk activities.

delusions—false, fixed, odd, or unusual beliefs about external reality that are not accepted by other members of the person's culture or subculture, yet are firmly sustained despite clear evidence to the contrary

hallucinations—sensory perceptions (seeing, hearing, feeling, and smelling) in the absence of an outside stimulus

When patients experience mixed symptoms while hypomanic, they may not recognize these periods as distinct from a depressive period. Careful questioning is important to explore this possibility when considering the differential diagnosis.

Feedback from family and friends helps the clinician distinguish between abnormal elevations of mood and the person's baseline levels of energy, goal-directed behavior, and personality. Hypomania is an abnormal change from usual behavior and not merely a good or happy mood.

Recognizing Symptoms of Depression

A **major depressive episode** is characterized by depressed mood or loss of interest or pleasure in previously enjoyed activities for a period of at least two weeks. Additionally, the individual may experience some or all of the following:

- Increased or decreased need for sleep
- Increased or decreased appetite
- Loss of energy
- Difficulty initiating action/behavior
- Diminished ability to concentrate
- Social withdrawal
- Feelings of worthlessness
- Thoughts of suicide or death

In children and adolescents, the predominant mood may be irritable rather than sad, accompanied by additional symptoms from the preceding list.

When they are depressed, people with bipolar disorder are often in a profoundly sad, irritable, or "numb" mood. They may report that life is totally without pleasure and not worth living, despite acknowledging positive things that "should" help them feel happy or satisfied. During depression, people lose interest and enjoyment in their usual activities, including basic pleasures such as eating and sex. Many people with depression experience hopelessness and can't imagine that they will ever feel better.

Core depression symptoms are changes in sleeping and eating habits. Many find it difficult to fall asleep, waking up several times each night and earlier in the morning than desired. About 20 percent of depressed people sleep more than they normally do. In all cases, people experiencing depression report that they don't feel rested even after adequate sleep. They may also experience changes in appetite. While some individuals lose weight, others experience an appetite increase, without necessarily feeling that the food they eat is satisfying or appealing.

Persons with depression often have difficulty with concentration, memory, and decision making. There is impairment in the person's social and/or occupational functioning.

Recognizing a Mixed Episode

A **mixed episode** is characterized by a period of at least one week in which the criteria are met both for a manic episode and for a major depressive episode nearly every day. The individual may experience rapidly alternating moods (sadness, irritability, euphoria) accompanied by symptoms of a manic episode and a major depressive episode.

The experience of clinically significant depression goes far beyond an everyday sad feeling.

Untreated, lengthy periods of severe depression can lead to thoughts about or actual attempts to commit suicide, making treatment particularly critical for those with bipolar disorder.

See pages 25–26 for a discussion of suicide assessment.

What Are the Criteria for Diagnosing Bipolar Disorder?

The potential diagnoses for someone experiencing alternating mood states include the following (APA, 2000):

- ▶ **Bipolar I Disorder (BDI)**—Patients meet the criteria for at least one lifetime **full manic episode**; most patients experience depressive episodes as well.

- ▶ **Bipolar II Disorder (BDII)**—Patients experience both hypomanic and depressive episode(s). Most patients predominantly experience depression with occasional hypomanic symptoms or mood lability.

- ▶ **Cyclothymic Disorder**—Patients experience numerous periods of both **hypomanic** and **depressive** symptoms over a two-year period without meeting criteria for full episodes of either.

- ▶ **Bipolar Disorder Not Otherwise Specified (BD NOS)**—Patients have cyclic moods and other symptoms consistent with bipolar disorder, but do not meet the criteria for any of the other three diagnoses.

Figure 2.2 indicates episode types (major depressive, manic, hypomanic, or mixed) that are characteristic for each diagnosis along with a summary of *DSM–IV–TR* criteria. The term "subthreshold symptoms" indicates that the symptoms are not strong enough to meet *DSM* criteria for a full mood episode by either severity and/or duration.

Diagnostic Specifiers for Bipolar I Disorder and Bipolar II Disorder

DSM–IV–TR explicitly endorses more detailed *specifiers* for bipolar disorder. These specifiers impact the treatment response and illness course for many patients.

For manic and depressive episodes, specifiers of the current clinical status and/or features include the following:

- ▶ Mild, moderate, severe symptoms without psychotic features/severe with psychotic features
- ▶ Chronic
- ▶ With *catatonic features*
- ▶ With *melancholic features*
- ▶ With *atypical features*
- ▶ With postpartum onset

During a manic episode, about half of all patients experience psychotic symptoms. These symptoms in bipolar disorder may

Individuals with BDI must meet criteria for at least one manic or mixed episode in their lifetime.

See Appendix A for a reprint of corresponding DSM–IV–TR criteria.

Bipolar diagnoses refer to lifetime history of mood episodes. Once an individual meets criteria for Bipolar II disorder (at least one episode each of hypomania and major depression), he or she is never again diagnosed with Bipolar NOS. Similarly, a person who has experienced a manic episode (BDI) cannot revert to a diagnosis of BDII or BD-NOS, even if much of their clinical course is depressive with hypomanic symptoms.

specifiers—*DSM–IV*-defined categories for specific symptoms that may occur with bipolar disorder such as psychotic or atypical symptoms

catatonic features—clinical features characterized by marked psychomotor disturbance that may involve immobility, excessive motor activity, extreme negativism, inability or refusal to speak, peculiar voluntary movements or speech

melancholic features—loss of interest or pleasure in all or almost all activities and lack of reactivity to usually pleasurable stimuli

Figure 2.2   Linking Bipolar Diagnostic Criteria with Depressive, Manic, Hypomanic, and Mixed Episodes

Episodes Associated with Bipolar Disorder	BDI	BDII	Cyclothymia	Bipolar Disorder NOS
Major Depressive Episode Characteristics • Depressed mood • At least two weeks' duration • Loss of interest or pleasure • Irritable mood rather than sad (in children) • Changes in appetite, weight, sleep, or psychomotor activity • Decreased energy • Feelings of worthlessness or guilt • Difficulty concentrating or making decisions • Recurrent thoughts of death or suicide		X	Subthreshold Symptoms	Subthreshold Symptoms
Manic Episode Characteristics • Persistently elevated, expansive, or irritable mood • At least one week's duration (or less if hospitalization is required) • Inflated self-esteem or grandiosity • Decreased need for sleep • Pressured speech • Flight of ideas • Distractibility • Increased involvement in goal-directed activities or psychomotor agitation • Excessive involvement in pleasurable and high-risk activities	X			
Hypomanic Episode Characteristics • Persistently elevated, expansive, or irritable mood • At least four days' duration • Inflated self-esteem or grandiosity • Decreased need for sleep • Pressured speech • Flight of ideas • Distractibility • Increased involvement in goal-directed activities or psychomotor agitation • Excessive involvement in pleasurable and high-risk activities		X	Subthreshold Symptoms	Subthreshold Symptoms
Mixed Episode Characteristics • Criteria met both for a manic episode and for a major depressive episode nearly every day during at least a 1-week period • The mood disturbance is sufficiently severe to cause significant distress or impairment in functioning.	X			

be indistinguishable from psychotic symptoms experienced by patients with schizophrenia, including delusions, hallucinations, *tangentiality*, *derailment*, and other signs of cognitive disorganization.

Course Specifiers

In addition to the preceding specifiers, for patients who are **not currently** in a manic, hypomanic, or depressed state, the clinician can specify if the person is in partial or full remission. For all active diagnoses, the clinician has the option to describe some characteristics of the typical course of illness for that individual:

- ▸ Longitudinal course (with or without interepisode recovery)—this is an opportunity to indicate formally whether the person tends to have periods of relative wellness between mood episodes.
- ▸ With *seasonal pattern*—this specifier gives the clinician an opportunity to indicate whether the patient's depressive symptoms coincide predictably with a season of the year. Recent evidence suggests that there may also be a seasonal component for hypomania and mania (Suppes et al., 2001).
- ▸ With rapid cycling—this specifier is used to indicate whether the person tends to experience four or more episodes in each year.

Of these, the rapid cycling specifier is most commonly used, as there is accumulating evidence that those with rapid cycling are more difficult to treat (Calabrese et al., 2005; Kupka et al., 2003; Kupka et al., 2005; Schneck et al., 2008). In some cases, persons with rapid cycling may experience chronic and persistent symptoms with little to no intermittent periods of euthymia.

What Tools Exist for Diagnosing Bipolar Disorder?

There is no simple diagnostic tool, such as a blood test, to assess for the presence of bipolar disorder. Trained mental health providers conduct clinical interviews and may administer self-report or clinician-rated scales to assess for symptom presence and severity.

This section reviews medical assessment and clinical interviewing (including collecting family psychiatric history) and lists symptom scales used for evaluation—clinician-administered, self-report, and general psychiatric tools. Appendix B presents detailed information on each of the symptom evaluation scales listed in this chapter.

atypical features—mood reactivity and at least two of the following: increased appetite or weight gain, excessive sleep, the sensation that one's limbs are too heavy to move, and a long-standing pattern of sensitivity to perceived interpersonal rejection

tangentiality—speech characterized by giving unrelated answers to direct questions and frequently changing the topic

derailment—quality of speech characterized by loose associations or an inability to stay on topic; sequential connection between ideas, which are difficult or impossible to follow because the person wanders to relatively or totally unrelated subjects

seasonal pattern—onset and remission of depressive symptoms occur at characteristic times of the year

Conducting a Medical Assessment

Since bipolar disorder is a clinical syndrome caused by brain dysfunction, it is important to rule out physiological causes for the symptoms. The *DSM–IV–TR* recognizes the potential of medical problems causing clinical symptoms under the diagnosis "Mood Disorder due to a General Medical Condition."

Some physiological causes to consider are the following:

embolic stroke—a type of ischemic stroke that occurs when a blood clot or a cholesterol plaque travels into the brain and blocks an artery

▶ **Embolic stroke**, which occurs typically in an elderly individual. For example, parietal lobe strokes have been implicated in both the development of depression and mania for some individuals. The parietal lobe is the brain lobe sitting behind the frontal cortex on each side of the midline.

▶ **Thyroid conditions** including **hyperthyroidism** (an excess of thyroid hormone), which can cause manic-like symptoms, or **hypothyroidism** (decreased thyroid hormone), which can cause depression-like symptoms. Blood tests will indicate changes in hormone levels.

Both conditions are associated with physical symptoms not usually observed in patients with bipolar disorder (e.g., elevated heart rate and blood pressure in hyperthyroidism and sensitivity to temperature change as well as skin bruises in hypothyroidism).

Research has also shown that the abuse of some drugs, including cocaine and steroids, can produce bipolar-like symptoms.

▶ **Temporal lobe epilepsy**, which is associated with many of the same symptoms that can be seen in bipolar disorder—no coincidence since one of the brain structures implicated in bipolar disorder is the temporal lobe.

▶ **Neoplastic or cancer syndromes**, which have also been associated with some patients' change in usual presentation and development of bipolar-like symptoms.

From the Patient's Perspective

My boss called me in today and was concerned that my work didn't seem to be as complete as a month or two ago. My co-workers are also complaining that I don't follow through on team projects these days. I know something is strange since I only sleep four hours a night. It's just so nice to have all this energy! When the credit card bill came today, my husband went through the roof; $700 in online purchases just in the last week. Maybe I should see a psychiatrist again, just to get everyone off my back.

Past history of head injuries should always be part of a medical assessment for bipolar disorder because head injury in and of itself can either cause or aggravate bipolar symptoms. Given that many untreated patients with bipolar disorder have low impulse control and a tendency to engage in risky behavior, the possibility for head injury becomes particularly pertinent.

When an individual is first seen with mood symptoms, the physician should conduct a physical and neurological assessment, including blood work that includes baseline chemistries and thyroid function, to assess for the possibility of these physiological disorders.

Although brain tumors and arterial-venous malformations are rare causes of bipolar disorder symptoms, physicians should consider a brain scan for those patients for whom one has never been conducted.

Conducting the Clinical Interview

A thorough clinical interview is an invaluable part of the assessment process. The interview provides a framework for understanding results of other assessment tools, such as questionnaires, as well as an opportunity to develop rapport and observe the patient's behavior, *affect*, and reactions to life events.

affect—the external expression of emotion

Clinical interviews can vary in the amount of structure provided. Most include some questions related to the patient's strengths, goals, nature and history of the problem, diagnosis, and relevant personal and family history. Although not comprehensive, the clinical areas covered in the checklist in Figure 2.3 can help with diagnosis and treatment planning.

Using Structured Symptom Evaluation Tools

Symptom evaluation tools clarify diagnoses and include structured clinical interviews, clinician-administered observational rating scales, self-ratings, and general assessments of psychiatric symptoms.

Appendix B includes detailed information on specific tools, including suicide assessment measures.

Structured Clinical Interviews

Highly structured diagnostic interviews were developed to reduce the emphasis on clinician judgment present in open-ended interviews. These interviews may require specialized training to administer correctly and can be time consuming. However, they have the benefit of providing more specific and objective criteria for diagnostic decisions. Some examples include the following (Endicott & Spitzer, 1978; First, Spitzer,

Figure 2.3   Clinical Interview Checklist

	Assessment Topics	Rationale
Problem History	• Description of symptoms, including extent to which they disrupt/disturb ability to function • Initial onset of symptoms • Intensity and duration of symptoms consistent with hypomania, mania, and depression • Changes in frequency or character of symptoms over time • Antecedents/consequences of symptoms • History of prior treatment/attempts to resolve symptoms	To gain insight into the course of illness for the individual, increase motivation for treatment, and target new treatment approaches in which the patient may be more compliant
Personal/Developmental Background	• Infancy—developmental milestones, early medical history • Family atmosphere, characterization of family of origin, relationships • School adjustment and performance • Medical history • Family history of psychiatric illness and treatment response, including any history of suicide	To help identify family history of any mood or other psychiatric disorders, distinguish medical factors that may be important, identify the degree to which symptoms may have impacted academic performance, and target educational needs to enable the patient to become an informed participant in treatment
Relationships	• Interpersonal relationships over time • Relationship/marriage history • Current social supports • Description of current living situation, relationships	To help assess the type and degree of social support available to the individual as well as the extent to which symptoms may have impaired the ability to engage in fulfilling and successful personal relationships
Financial/Occupational Background	• Work history • Current work status, performance, and satisfaction • Career goals • Economic stability	To help assess the difference between work reality, function, and goals. Those living with economic instability have additional pressures that may impact response to treatment; this pressure may add to depressive symptoms or foster choices inconsistent with treatment, like working several jobs around the clock.
Miscellaneous/Other	• Fears, concerns, worries • Self-concept • Social/recreational activities/outlets • History of legal problems • Drug and/or alcohol use	To learn important goals/concerns of the patient. Additionally, information about history may confirm past symptom severity (e.g., accumulating huge financial debt and lawsuits due to gambling while manic). Current use of drugs and/or alcohol can negatively impact the course of the disorder and treatment response.

Gibbon, & Williams, 1997; Robins, Marcus, Reich, Cunningham, & Gallagher, 1996):

▶ The Schedule for Affective Disorders and Schizophrenia (SADS)

▶ Diagnostic Interview Schedule (DIS)

▶ The Structured Clinical Interview for the *DSM–IV* (SCID)

Clinician-Administered Observational Rating Scales

Many assessment tools combine structured to semistructured interviews with behavioral observations. A trained interviewer conducts the face-to-face interviews and rates discrete symptom domains. These instruments incorporate information obtained through behavioral observations and in some cases collateral information, such as reports from family members, close friends, or other clinicians. There are many published scales to measure symptoms of **hypomania and mania**. Some of the most commonly used scales include the following (Altman, Hedeker, Janicak, Peterson, & Davis, 1994; Young, Biggs, Ziegler, & Mayer, 1978):

▶ Young Mania Rating Scale (YMRS)

▶ Clinician Administered Rating Scale for Mania (CARS-M)

There are many published scales to measure symptoms of **depression**. Some of the most commonly used scales include the following (Davidson et al., 1986; Hamilton, 1960, 1967; Kearns et al., 1982; Montgomery & Äsberg, 1979; Rush, Giles et al., 1986; Rush, Trivedi et al., 2003; Williams, 1988):

▶ Inventory of Depressive Symptomatology—Clinician-Rated (IDS-C)

▶ Quick Inventory of Depressive Symptomatology-Clinical Rated (QIDS-C)

▶ Hamilton Rating Scale for Depression (HAM-D) and the structured interview companion to the instrument

▶ Montgomery-Äsberg Depression Rating Scale (MADRS)

Self-Ratings

Patients can report their own symptoms using self-report, pencil-and-paper symptom inventories. These tools are appropriate for those patients who have *insight* and awareness of small but significant changes in mood, energy or sleep that may reliably precipitate a mood episode. Self ratings are not appropriate for patients who:

insight—understanding or awareness of one's mental or emotional condition

▶ Are not forthcoming with information

▶ Have limited insight into their symptoms and illness

▶ Are severely ill and possibly unable to accurately complete these self-administered reports

▶ Have problems with extensive reading or other language barriers

Self-report instruments developed specifically for comprehensive reporting of bipolar disorder symptoms are the following (Bauer et al., 1991; Denicoff et al., 2000; Hirschfeld et al., 2000; Leverich & Post, 1998; Post, Roy-Byrne, & Uhde, 1998):

See Appendix C for a sample log from the Life Chart.

▶ The Life Chart Method

▶ The Internal State Scale (ISS)

Additionally, the Mood Disorder Questionnaire (MDQ) is a brief, self-report **diagnostic** instrument that screens for symptoms consistent with a bipolar disorder diagnosis (Hirschfeld et al., 2003). A new version of the MDQ, MDQ-Expanded, screens for current symptoms of mania, depression, and alcohol abuse (Hirschfeld & Compact Clinicals, 2005). These tools are a useful starting place in the diagnostic process, but they cannot alone reliably identify the presence of a bipolar disorder.

Other self-report tools measure either hypomania/mania or depression independently. Some of the more commonly used tools include the following (Altman, Hedeker, Peterson, & Davis, 1997; Beck, Steer, & Brown, 1986; Beck, Steer, & Garbin, 1988; Rush, Giles et al., 1986; Rush, Gullion, Basco, Jarrett, & Trivedi, 1996):

▶ The Altman Mania Rating Scale (AMRS)

▶ The Inventory for Depressive Symptoms-Self Report (IDS-SR) and the Quick Inventory for Depressive Symptoms-Self Report (QIDS-SR)

▶ The Beck Depression Inventory (BDI-2)

General Psychiatric Symptom Assessment Tools

A trained clinician might also choose to use a general measure of psychiatric symptoms and/or personality function to assist in the diagnostic process. These tools can help pinpoint other psychiatric symptoms that can co-occur with symptoms of mania and depression. Alternatively, there are many high-quality published interviews and self-report instruments that assess symptoms of psychosis, anxiety, anger, somatization, and other psychiatric symptoms that may be helpful to include in individual assessments as needed.

Although the following measures are not specific to symptoms of bipolar disorder, they can be helpful in differentiating presenting symptoms from those consistent with other disorders (Butcher, Dahlstrom, Graham, Tellegen, & Kaemmer, 1989; Millon, Davis,

& Millon, 1997; Overall & Gorham, 1998; Ventura, Nuechterlein, Subotnik, & Gilbert, 1995):

▶ The Brief Psychiatric Rating Scale (BPRS)

▶ The Minnesota Multiphasic Personality Inventory-2nd Edition (MMPI)

▶ The Millon Clinical Multiaxial Inventory (MCMI)

Appendix B offers information on specific tools, including suicide assessment measures.

Assessing Suicide Risk

Bipolar disorder is accompanied by a high risk for self-injury and suicide when untreated or when patients experience limited response to treatment (Baldessarini & Tondo, 2008; Tondo et al., 2003). Those with co-occurring alcohol or substance abuse or dependence are at greater risk for suicide, as are those who have made previous suicide attempts. Assessment of suicide risk is a complex and multidimensional task and should be an ongoing aspect of interactions between care providers and the patient.

There are multiple assessment tools designed to assist clinicians in assessing suicide risk. Most of these include some assessment of these general domains:

▶ The wish to live or die

▶ Experience of impulses related to suicide as well as control over these impulses

▶ Duration and frequency of suicidal ideation (thoughts)

▶ Specificity of ideas or plans for suicide

▶ Access to lethal means

▶ Any active preparation for suicide (e.g., writing letters to loved ones, giving away possessions)

▶ Deterrents to suicide (e.g., support from family members, family or pets dependent on the patient, or spiritual/religious beliefs)

In addition to assessing general domains, the clinician must consider the context in which these thoughts are occurring. The severity of depression, anger, impulsivity, use of drugs or alcohol, events in the person's life, and other variables must all be considered when evaluating the risk for suicide.

Following are descriptions of some assessment tools that may be helpful in routine clinical assessment of suicide risk.

▶ **Beck Scale for Suicide Ideation (BSS; self-administered version)**—The BSS is a 21-item self-report scale that is completed independently by the patient. Higher scores indicate increasing suicidal ideation and risk. As this scale takes about five to 10 minutes to complete, it can be useful as part of a package of assessment tools completed prior to routine visits. However, it should not substitute for face-to-face assessment of recent suicidal thoughts or plans.

▶ **Scale for Suicide Ideation (SSI; clinician-administered version)**—The SSI is administered in an approximately 10-minute interview with a clinician and

Collected retrospectively, the SSI results are subject to some bias, depending on the length of elapsed time or other factors that may obscure memory of the event.

can assess either current ideation or worst ideation ever experienced. It includes the same 21 items contained on the self-report version, the Beck Scale for Suicide Ideation, described above. The SSI provides a reliable, valid, and rapid method of systematically estimating suicidal ideation.

▶ **Suicide Intent Scale (SIS)**—The SIS is designed to measure the intensity of the attempter's wish to die at the time of the attempt and is typically administered to an individual after a suicide attempt. This scale has primarily been used in research settings, although the intensity of the person's wish to die is viewed as an important risk factor for future suicide attempts. The SIS includes 20 items, and it is administered by a trained clinician in a brief interview.

▶ **Beck Hopelessness Scale (BHS)**—The BHS is a 20-item true-false scale that can be completed independently by the patient in five to 10 minutes. Hopelessness correlates with the overall severity of depression and may be more related to risk for suicide than other symptoms of depression. Higher scores on the BHS, suggesting greater hopelessness, are associated with eventual suicide attempt or completion (Beck, Brown, Berchick, Stewart, & Steer, 1990; Beck, Steer, Kovacs, & Garrison, 1985). Hopelessness is not related to immediate risk, but rather risk over time. Fortunately, scores on the BHS decrease with successful treatment for depression (Beck et al., 1985).

Hopelessness is an indirect measure of suicidality, as those with greater pessimism about the future may be at greater risk for suicide.

What Differentiates Bipolar Disorder from Other Disorders?

Bipolar disorder is very likely to coexist with other psychiatric conditions. The presence of other psychiatric conditions increases the complexity of treatment and reduces the likelihood of symptom remission. Given the susceptibility of patients with bipolar disorder to become manic (BDI) or hypomanic (BDII) with use of certain medications, a careful balancing and monitoring of medications is often required. For example, if an antidepressant or stimulant medication is added to improve energy and goal-directed behavior, a patient with BDI must be on adequate antimanic treatment to avoid a risk of new manic symptoms.

When diagnosing bipolar disorder, the clinician must rule out the possibility that the individual's symptoms are related to:

▶ Major Depressive Disorder

▶ Substance-Induced Mood Disorder

- ▶ Mood Disorder due to a General Medical Condition
- ▶ Attention Deficit Hyperactivity Disorder
- ▶ Psychotic Disorders
- ▶ Anxiety Disorders

Major Depressive Disorder (MDD)—The most challenging differential diagnosis for clinicians is distinguishing bipolar disorder from unipolar depression, particularly in patients who experience hypomania and not mania (BDII). Patients may not recognize or correctly label periods of hypomania, particularly mixed hypomania. Thorough questioning of the individual and/or family or other collateral informants regarding lifetime occurrence of one or more episodes of hypomania or mania will resolve this issue. In addition to the depressive episode that is apparent in the presumed diagnosis of MDD, if there is a history of at least one manic episode, the patient meets criteria for bipolar I disorder. If there is a history of hypomania, criteria for BDII are met.

Many patients request help during depressive episodes, and if not queried specifically, clinicians may miss the history of hypomania or mania.

Substance-Induced Mood Disorder—A substance-induced mood disorder is a significant mood disturbance caused by the use of a substance (e.g., a drug of abuse, alcohol, a medication, or exposure to a toxin). Use or withdrawal from substances such as cocaine, amphetamines, or alcohol may produce symptoms similar to mania and/or depression, and these episodes should be described as a substance-induced mood disorder.

The clinician should specifically ask the patient about the onset of symptoms and the use of substances. For example, intoxication from cocaine may mimic a manic episode and would be described as a cocaine-induced mood disorder with manic features, according to *DSM–IV–TR* criteria. If mood symptoms do not remit after withdrawal of the substance and an appropriate time interval, the diagnosis of a bipolar disorder should be reconsidered.

When substance-induced mood disorder is suspected, appropriate laboratory tests and screenings should be performed to determine the exact etiology of mood symptoms.

Mood Disorder Due to a General Medical Condition—This diagnosis is reserved for mood symptoms judged to be a direct physiological consequence of a specific general medical condition. Certain medical conditions (e.g., brain tumor, Cushing's syndrome, or hypothyroidism) can mimic symptoms of either mania or depression. This determination can be made by a thorough medical history, laboratory findings, and physical examination.

Generally, if a patient is nonresponsive to treatments for bipolar disorder, the clinician should reconsider the diagnosis and perform further diagnostic tests to rule out other causes or contributing medical factors.

Physiological conditions that can produce bipolar-like symptoms include:

► Embolic stroke

► A hyperthyroid or a hypothyroid condition

► Temporal lobe epilepsy

► Neoplastic or cancer syndromes

► Abuse of some drugs, including cocaine and steroids

► Head injuries

Attention Deficit Hyperactivity Disorder (ADHD)—
ADHD must be differentiated from hypomania or mania, as they share the characteristics of impulsivity, poor judgment, and excessive activity. This differentiation is best accomplished by obtaining a thorough developmental history. Consider ADHD if:

► Symptoms of inattention, hyperactivity, or impulsivity consistently occurred prior to the age of 7 years.

► Early school history is characterized by persistent teacher complaints of such behaviors and disruption in learning.

Unlike other mood or psychotic disorders, ADHD can be diagnosed as a co-occurring condition in those with bipolar disorder.

ADHD is also characterized by a chronic course, while bipolar symptoms tend to be more **episodic**. Additionally, those with bipolar disorder have specific mood symptoms, such as sustained episodes of significant depression, which may or may not be present in those with ADHD.

Psychotic Disorders—Psychotic disorders and BDI can share a number of symptoms, including grandiose and persecutory delusions, irritability, depression, withdrawal, and agitation. This overlap is most pronounced early in the course of all disorders, before full symptoms of the disorder are present. However, diagnosis of all the psychotic disorders requires the presence of psychotic symptoms in the absence of prominent mood symptoms. In bipolar disorder, psychotic symptoms will occur with mood symptoms during the course of either depressive or manic episodes. Other areas that may help differentiate diagnoses are the type of accompanying symptoms, previous course, and family psychiatric history.

Psychotic disorders include schizoaffective disorder, schizophrenia, schizophreniform disorder, delusional disorder, and psychotic disorder not otherwise specified.

Anxiety Disorders—The prominent clinical presentation in multiple anxiety disorders is chronic and debilitating anxiety, versus fluctuating mood episodes on the bipolar spectrum. Persons with anxiety disorders present as chronically worried or fearful, and they have corresponding reductions in their ability to function as a result of those fears.

It is possible to have a diagnosis of both bipolar disorder and an anxiety disorder. In fact, bipolar disorder and anxiety disorders are highly associated. In a large epidemiological sample, a significant percentage of those with BDI and BDII had some lifetime anxiety disorder diagnosis (Merikangas et al., 2007). Therefore, the critical issue is not necessarily in differentiating bipolar symptoms from anxiety, but rather in determining whether coexisting anxiety symptoms may be present and require clinical attention as well.

Anxiety disorders include:

► Acute stress disorder

► Agoraphobia without history of panic disorder

► Anxiety disorder due to general medical condition

► Generalized anxiety disorder

► Obsessive-compulsive disorder

► Panic disorder with agoraphobia

► Panic disorder without agoraphobia

► Post-traumatic stress disorder

► Specific phobia

► Social phobia

► Substance-induced anxiety disorder

► Anxiety disorder NOS

How Does Bipolar Disorder Present in Children and Adolescents?

Symptoms of bipolar disorder may be difficult to recognize in children and adolescents, as they can be mistaken for age-appropriate emotions and behaviors. Symptoms of mania and depression may appear in a variety of behaviors. When manic, children and adolescents, in contrast to adults, are more likely to be irritable and prone to destructive outbursts than to be elated or euphoric. When depressed, there may be complaints of headaches, stomachaches, tiredness, poor school performance, poor communication, and extreme sensitivity to rejection or failure.

Treating bipolar disorder in children relies on experience in treating adults with the illness, since very few studies have been done of the effectiveness and safety of the medications currently used for adults when given to children and adolescents. Pediatric treatment guidelines for bipolar disorder have been generated based on available evidence and expert consensus (McClellan et al., 2007).

According to the American Academy of Child and Adolescent Psychiatry, up to one-third of the 3.4 million children and adolescents with depression in the United States may actually be experiencing the early onset of bipolar disorder.

Key Concepts for Chapter 2

1. Thorough assessment for the historical presence of hypomanic or manic symptoms is essential in differentiating bipolar disorder from unipolar depression.

2. Bipolar disorder is characterized by episodes of depression, hypomania, and for some individuals, mania. When individuals experience a full episode of mania and depression at the same time, the episode is referred to as "mixed."

3. Individuals with untreated bipolar disorder or those unresponsive to treatment are at increased risk for suicide.

4. In the *DSM–IV–TR*, recognized diagnoses for bipolar disorders include BDI, BDII, BD NOS, and cyclothymic disorder.

5. Rapid cycling is specified when the person experiences four or more episodes in a year. These patients may be less responsive to treatment.

6. There are many options and approaches to assessing bipolar disorder, including medical evaluation, clinical interview, and structured symptom assessments.

7. Other disorders can cause "bipolar-like" symptoms. It is important to differentiate bipolar disorder from major depressive disorder, substance-induced mood disorder, mood disorder due to a medical condition, and ADHD as well as psychotic and anxiety disorders.

Chapter 3
Biological Treatment of Bipolar Disorder

This chapter answers the following questions:

▶ **What Medications Have Received Approval from the Food and Drug Administration for Treatment of Bipolar Disorders?**—This section covers those medications that have received approval from the Food and Drug Administration for specific use in patients with bipolar disorder diagnoses.

▶ **What Are Treatment Guidelines for Bipolar Disorder?**—This section discusses the development and use of structured treatment guidelines for bipolar disorder.

▶ **What Medications Are Used to Treat Mania/Hypomania in Patients with Bipolar Disorder?**—This section covers medications for mania and hypomania, including treatment strategies and efficacy as well as using combination medications.

▶ **What Medications Are Used to Treat Depression in Patients with Bipolar Disorder?**—This section covers medications for depression, including treatment strategies and efficacy.

▶ **What Strategies Are Recommended for Maintenance Treatment?**—This section provides information on treatments that are effective for the maintenance treatment of patients with bipolar disorder.

▶ **How Can Medication Treatment of Side Effects Be Managed?**—This section presents strategies for treating the side effects sometimes experienced with medication treatment.

▶ **How Are Electroconvulsive Therapy (ECT) and Alternative Medicine Used to Treat Patients with Bipolar Disorder?**—This section discusses electroconvulsive therapy (ECT) and other alternative approaches.

▶ **How Does the Presence of Co-Occurring Disorders Impact Medication Treatment for Bipolar Disorder?**—This section addresses the impact of co-occurring disorders on medication treatment strategies.

A LTHOUGH there is no cure for bipolar disorder, in most cases it can be treated and controlled with medication. Treatment options have increased significantly over the past 30 years beyond lithium, which was the primary treatment option for bipolar disorder until the 1980s. While lithium is helpful for both depressive and hypomanic/manic symptoms, other medications are also effective for treating mood states. For example, the anticonvulsant valproate is a mainstay of treatment for mood instability with other anticonvulsants having more specific benefits. A productive area of newer research focuses on the extent to which bipolar disorder symptoms may be successfully treated with the second-generation antipsychotic medications (e.g., aripiprazole, asenapine, clozapine, olanzapine, quetiapine, risperidone, or ziprasidone). Although individuals diagnosed with bipolar disorder require lifetime monitoring

Our increasing knowledge and understanding of brain function leads to better and more specific drug development. Observing responses to specific medications likewise informs us regarding brain function and processes.

*It is important to note that **all medication use** must balance benefits and risks for each individual patient.*

and treatment, many can achieve and maintain stable moods for long periods.

Most of our knowledge about medication treatment for bipolar disorder comes from research in bipolar I disorder (BDI). However, in recent years there has been more attention given to bipolar II disorder and ways in which treatment may differ for these individuals. Bipolar II disorder (BDII) is an important diagnostic group that is estimated to be as common as bipolar I disorder. In some ways, those with bipolar II disorder may be more challenging to treat, as they may not recognize hypomanic symptoms, or while they acknowledge them as different from usual behavior, they perceive them to be beneficial and avoid treatment. Others are misdiagnosed with major depressive disorder and/or experience persistent depressive episodes (Suppes & Dennehy, 2002). There are many treatment options for those with bipolar II disorder, but only one medication (quetiapine) has been studied sufficiently in this population to warrant Food and Drug Administration (FDA) indication for treatment of these individuals.

As many as 50 percent of patients with BDI experience psychotic symptoms during manic or mixed episodes. However, these symptoms are viewed as part of the illness and in most cases respond to antimanic treatments, including lithium and anticonvulsants with antimanic properties. Therefore, this text does not specifically address treatment of psychosis in bipolar disorder.

Published guidelines for the treatment of bipolar disorder include the Canadian Network for Mood and Anxiety Treatments (CANMAT) and International Society for Bipolar Disorder (ISBD) Collaborative Guideline, Texas Implementation of Medication Algorithms (TIMA) guidelines, American Psychiatric Association Guidelines, Veterans Administration Guideline, and the Expert Consensus Guideline (VA, DoD, 2010; Hirschfeld et al., 2002; Keck, Perlis, & Otto, 2004; Suppes, Dennehy et al., 2005; Yatham et al., 2009).

What Medications Have Received Approval from the Food and Drug Administration for Treatment of Bipolar Disorders?

The Food and Drug Administration (FDA) requires drug manufacturers to establish certain goals for effectiveness and safety before providing an "indication" that a drug is recommended for a specific use. In the last 10 years, the number of indications for treatment of different phases of illness in bipolar disorder has grown substantially, supporting more options for clinicians and patients. Table 3.1 presents the medications that have received an indication from the FDA for treatment of symptoms of bipolar disorder. In some cases those indications are for monotherapy, while in others the recommendation is to use the compound in combination with lithium or valproate. Generic and trade names for commonly used medications are presented in Figure 3.1.

Table 3.1   Summary of Compounds with FDA Indications for Treatment of Bipolar Disorder

Drug Name	Bipolar I Disorder			Maintenance	Bipolar II
	Acute Mania	Acute Mixed Episodes	Acute Depression		
Lithium ("Li")	X			X	
Valproate ("VPA")	X				
Carbamazepine ("CBZ")	X*	X*			
Lamotrigine				X	
Aripiprazole	X	X		X	
Olanzapine	X	X	X	X	
Risperidone	X	X			
Risperidone long-acting injectable				X	
Asenapine	X	X			
Quetiapine and Quetiapine XR	X	X*	X	X	X
Ziprasidone	X	X		X	
Olanzapine and fluoxetine HCl			X		

*Extended release version only
Note: FDA indication may be for monotherapy, combination use (with either Li or DVP), or both. Please see the PDR for exact recommendations.

What Are Treatment Guidelines for Bipolar Disorder?

Medication *algorithms* and guidelines allow the clinician to apply a systematic approach to treatment, based on expert recommendations. Evidence-based algorithms for the treatment of bipolar disorder are available to guide clinical decision making. These can be helpful as they codify the evidence in support of widening sets of treatment options into hierarchical decision trees with wide latitude to make individual decisions based on patient history, preference, and medical concerns.

algorithms—an organized set of specific recommendations that are evidence-based, often informed by expert consensus opinion when there are inadequate studies to inform treatment decisions

What Medications Are Used to Treat Mania/Hypomania in Patients with Bipolar Disorder?

Medications for treating symptoms of mania/hypomania include lithium, anticonvulsants, and second-generation antipsychotic

Guidelines for diagnosis, assessment, and treatment of children with bipolar disorder were recently published by the American Academy of Child and Adolescent Psychiatry (McClellan, Kowatch, & Findling, 2007).

Figure 3.1   Trade Names for Common Bipolar Medications

Medication	Trade Name(s)	Medication	Trade Name(s)
Lithium	Eskalith,® Lithobid®		
Anticonvulsants			
Carbamazepine	Equetro,™ Tegretol,® Carbatrol®	Valproate	Depakote® Depakene®
Lamotrigine	Lamictal®		
Antidepressants			
Amitriptyline	Elavil,® Endep®	Maprotiline	Ludiomil®
Amoxapine	Ascendin®	Mirtazapine	Remeron®
Bupropion	Wellbutrin®	Nortriptyline	Aventyl,® Pamelor®
Citalopram	Celexa®	Paroxetine Phenelzine	Paxil® Nardil®
Clomipramine	Anafranil®	Protriptyline	Vivactil®
Desipramine	Norpramin®	Sertraline	Zoloft®
Desvenlafaxine	Pristiq®	Trazodone	Desyrel®
Doxepin	Adapin,® Sinequan®	Tranylcypromine	Parnate®
Duloxetine	Cymbalta®	Trimipramine	Surmontil®
Fluoxetine	Prozac®	Venlafaxine	Effexor®
Fluvoxamine	Luvox®		
Imipramine	Tofranil®		
Second-Generation Antipsychotics			
Aripiprazole	Abilify®	Olanzapine/Fluoxetine Combination	Geodon®
Asenapine	Clozaril®	Quetiapine	Risperdal® Risperdal Consta®
Clozapine	Saphris®	Risperidone	Seroquel® Seroquel XR®
Olanzapine	Zyprexa®	Ziprasidone	Symbyax®
MAOIs			
Isocarboxazid	Marplan®	Selegiline	Eldepryl®
Phenelzine	Nardil®	Tranylcypromine	Parnate®
Other			
Pramipexole	Mirapex		

drugs as well as combinations of medications across different drug classes. Although all of these medications act on the brain to decrease manic, mixed, or hypomanic symptoms (e.g., an antimanic effect), they each operate through distinct mechanisms of action. Complicated sets of checks and balances exist within cells, and it is likely that medications fundamentally work by decreasing or modifying cell activity, leading to cellular balance that minimizes altered behavior and clinical syndromes. For example, valproate (VPA) and carbamazepine (CBZ) are both anticonvulsants that decrease excessive excitability and enhance the brain's inhibitory functions responsible for providing checks and balances in brain cell activity. However, valproate also acts on calcium ionic channels and may impact secondary messenger systems differently than CBZ.

For comprehensive information about medications, clinicians should carefully review package inserts for individual medications or access the **Physicians' Desk Reference (PDR).**

Figure 3.2 summarizes recommended doses and more common side effects for each of the medications that are beneficial in treatment of mania, hypomania, and mixed states, compiled from the *Physicians' Desk Reference* and the scientific literature. These medications are helpful in returning brain function to more normalized states. As symptoms decrease, sleep increases, irritability decreases, moods are more even, and the patient is

Figure 3.2   Medication Dosages and Common Side Effects for Treating Acute Phase of Mania/Hypomania in Patients with Bipolar Disorder*

Type/Class: Medication	Usual Target Dose**	Usual Maximum Recommended Dose (level)	Recommended Administration Schedule	Common Side Effects***
Lithium	0.6–1.0 mEq/L	1.2 mEq/L	2 times daily or at bedtime	Tremor, drowsiness, nausea/vomiting, increased urine output, muscle weakness, thirst, dry mouth, cognitive impairment
Anticonvulsants:				
Valproate (Divalproex is the FDA-approved formulation for bipolar disorder)	70–80 µg/mL	125 ug/mL	2 times daily or at bedtime	Nausea/vomiting, increased appetite with weight gain, sedation, hair loss, reversible increases in liver function tests, reversible thrombocytopenia, rarely pancreatitis
Carbamazepine (carbamazepine-ERC**** is the FDA-approved formulation for bipolar disorder)	4–12 ug/mL 400–1600 mg/day	12 ug/mL 1600 mg/day	2 times daily	Dizziness, drowsiness, blurred vision, fatigue, nausea, vomiting, ataxia, tremor

(continued)

Figure 3.2 (*Continued*)

Type/Class: Medication	Usual Target Dose**	Usual Maximum Recommended Dose (level)	Recommended Administration Schedule	Common Side Effects***
Second-Generation Oral Antipsychotic Medications:				
Aripiprazole	15–30 mg/day	30 mg/day	Once daily	Sedation, Parkinson-like symptoms,***** internal feeling of restlessness or agitation (akathisia)
Asenapine	5–10 mg BID	10 mg BID	Twice a day	Sedation, somnolence, nausea, headache, weight gain, dizziness, akathisia
Clozapine	100–300 mg/day	900 mg/day	At bedtime	Sedation, weight gain, dry mouth, constipation, and potential mental confusion, orthostatic hypotension, rapid heart rate, excessive salivation, constipation, nausea, and vomiting
Olanzapine	10–15 mg/day	20 mg/day	2 times daily or at bedtime	Sedation, weight gain, dry mouth, constipation, and potential mental confusion, mild Parkinson-like symptoms,***** and slowed movements
Quetiapine	300–600 mg/day	800 mg/day	2 times daily or at bedtime	Sedation, orthostatic hypotension, weight gain, potential thyroid inhibition
Risperidone	2–4 mg/day	6 mg/day	2 times daily or at bedtime	Sedation, Parkinson-like symptoms,***** weight gain, hypotension, sexual dysfunction; elevated prolactin
Ziprasidone	120–160 mg/day	160 mg/day	2 times daily	Sedation, nausea and vomiting, constipation, Parkinson-like symptoms,***** dizziness

*This review of medications is intended to provide information on commonly used medications but not to be comprehensive. Additionally, this information is not intended to provide prescription information, and a physician or appropriate individual should be consulted prior to making medication changes. For full information about medications, physicians should carefully review package inserts for individual medications or access the *Physicians' Desk Reference*.

**Doses used for maintenance treatment may be lower.

***Side effects may be less with slow-absorbing forms of medications. Lithium, divalproex, carbamazepine, and quetiapine also available in slow-absorption (or extended-release) formulations.

****Therapeutic blood levels are not required for carbamazepine ERC.

***** These symptoms include flat facial expression, stiff muscles, and slowed movements.

able to concentrate and gradually resume usual activities. Prior to the use of medications, untreated mania was observed to last 6 to 10 weeks. Medication treatment minimizes symptoms in days, though full symptom resolution often requires three to four weeks.

Lithium—In 1970, lithium became the first drug to receive U.S. Food and Drug Administration (FDA) approval for the treatment of manic episodes in bipolar disorder. Later, it also received an indication for prevention of new episodes. Lithium remains an important option for treatment of bipolar disorders.

Anticonvulsants—A number of research results indicate that certain anticonvulsant medications are helpful for treating mania and/or mixed states, especially:

▶ Valproate (most research trials have studied divalproex, the enteric-coated form of valproate)

▶ Carbamazepine

Second-Generation Antipsychotic Medications—This group of medications represents a significant improvement in options for patients with schizophrenia and bipolar disorder. Unlike the "typical" or older antipsychotics, these medications (as a group) cause fewer, less severe, or no movement disorder side effects, such as dystonia, akathisia, and others. Several of these medications are available in extended release and injectable formulations that provide important alternatives for individual patients.

Testing for blood levels of lithium and some anticonvulsant medications helps ensure dosing within the recommended therapeutic range for treatment of bipolar disorder.

maintenance treatment— an ongoing treatment believed to prevent or minimize the development of new episodes of mania, depression, or mixed states

The second-generation antipsychotic medications which have antimanic properties include:

▶ Aripiprazole

▶ Asenapine

▶ Clozapine

▶ Olanzapine

▶ Risperidone

▶ Quetiapine

▶ Ziprasidone

While the antimanic properties of these medications have been evident for a number of years, an important new discovery is that some of these medications also decrease depressive symptoms when given to acutely depressed patients with bipolar disorder. See the section on treatment of depressive symptoms in bipolar disorder for more detail (page 42).

Current research with the second-generation antipsychotic agents focuses on developing usage guidelines, appropriate combination use for optimal results, linking specific agents with differing clinical symptom patterns, and addressing long-term safety and tolerance issues. Each of the medications listed in Figure 3.2 has a somewhat different impact on brain receptors. Thus, while one medication may be less effective in an individual, another medication from this class may be more effective due to differences in the following:

▶ How the medication changes activity of brain neurons or affects different brain receptors

▶ What side effects different patients experience

▶ The presence of co-existing psychiatric or other medical conditions

Effectiveness of Medications for Treating Mania/Hypomania Symptoms of Bipolar Disorder

Significant efficacy studies have been completed assessing the benefits of lithium, anticonvulsants, and second-generation antipsychotics. The following section focuses exclusively on medications with evidence for support of their use in treatment of hypomanic and manic symptoms.

Lithium

Controlled studies have demonstrated that lithium is superior to placebo for treatment of acute mania when prescribed for one to three weeks at a therapeutic level (Grunze, 2003). However, much of this early research has been criticized for methodological problems, particularly the reliance on *crossover designs*, many of which abruptly discontinued lithium for those in the placebo group—an approach that may, in itself, cause or exacerbate bipolar symptoms (Perlis et al., 2002; Suppes, Baldessarini, Faedda, & Tohen, 1991). Other data suggest that patients with mixed mania, or dysphoric mania, respond better to anticonvulsants than lithium; therefore, lithium is not the first choice for patients with mixed presentations (Swann et al., 1997).

Anticonvulsants

Research results indicate that valproate and carbamazepine are effective in treating hypomanic and manic symptoms in bipolar disorder.

Valproate—There are good, placebo-controlled data supporting this drug's efficacy as a single therapy for mania or mixed states (Bowden et al., 1994; Pope, McElroy, Keck, & Hudson, 1991). Divalproex sodium, the enteric-coated form of valproate, was approved by the FDA for the treatment of acute mania in the early 1990s. In head-to-head studies with lithium, divalproex was more effective in decreasing symptoms of mixed states (Swann et al., 1997).

crossover design—a type of clinical study in which patients are first randomized to one treatment arm; then at some point during the study they are "crossed over" to receive the other treatment option

Younger women may be at risk of developing polycystic ovarian syndrome and hyperandrogenism soon after beginning valproate treatment (Joffe et al., 2006; Rasgon et al., 2005). However, the risk may be lower than indicated in earlier, smaller studies (Isojarvi et al., 1993).

Carbamazepine—Similar to valproate, this medication may be particularly helpful when depressive symptoms are present during mania (Goodwin & Jamison, 2007). Placebo-controlled studies of the slow-absorbing form of carbamazepine support good effectiveness and tolerability for acute manic or mixed symptoms in bipolar disorder (Weisler, Hirschfeld et al., 2006; Weisler, Kalali, & Ketter, 2004). These recent placebo-controlled studies led to the FDA approval of carbamazipine (extended release) to treat acute manic or mixed states in patients with bipolar I disorder.

With carbamazepine, there are some concerns with drug interaction and tolerability (Suppes, Dennehy et al., 2005). These concerns can be addressed through careful management, such as monitoring blood levels and side effects. If using carbamazepine ERC, monitoring of blood levels to ensure dosing within the therapeutic range is not necessary.

Second-Generation Antipsychotics

Recent studies conducted under double-blind, placebo-controlled conditions have demonstrated the antimanic properties of aripiprazole, asenapine, olanzapine, quetiapine, risperidone, and ziprasidone.

Aripiprazole—This medication is effective for both manic and mixed episodes, demonstrated in two multicenter, randomized, double-blind, placebo-controlled studies (Keck, Marcus et al., 2003; Sachs et al., 2006).

Asenapine—In two randomized, controlled trials of asenapine monotherapy compared to placebo and olanzapine (total $n = 976$) and in one randomized, controlled trial of adjunctive therapy in adult patients with bipolar I disorder ($n = 318$), asenapine demonstrated significant reductions in symptoms of mania relative to placebo (McIntyre et al., 2008, 2009a,b). A double-blind extension study was available for patients who completed either of the two 3-week, double-blind trials (McIntyre et al., 2009b), in which those who received placebo were blindly switched to asenapine. Results suggest that asenapine and olanzapine performed similarly under these conditions.

Clozapine—Clozapine was the first second-generation antipsychotic. The finding that clozapine was helpful to severely ill patients with schizophrenia was the impetus for development of additional new antipsychotic medications. Although there have been no placebo-controlled studies of clozapine in bipolar disorder, an open, controlled, one-year study and open monotherapy in acute mania support efficacy (Calabrese et al., 1996; Suppes, Webb et al., 1999). Importantly, these studies and others included more

Clozapine is an antipsychotic that has a clearly defined role in the treatment of refractory bipolar disorder, both as monotherapy and in combination with other psychotropic medications (Frye et al., 1998; McElroy et al., 1991; Suppes, Webb et al., 1999).

severely ill, treatment-resistant patients with bipolar disorder. Clozapine is a potential treatment option for patients who have failed other treatments, who are compliant with the required monitoring, and who are free of contraindicated medical conditions.

Olanzapine—The effectiveness of this medication for reducing manic symptoms has been demonstrated in placebo-controlled and double-blind trials (Berk, Ichim, & Brook, 1999; Tohen, Jacobs et al., 2000; Tohen, Sanger et al., 1999). Olanzapine in combination with either lithium or valproate is also indicated for the treatment of manic symptoms (Tohen et al., 2002).

There are concerns over sustained use of olanzapine due to safety and tolerability issues, particularly related to weight gain and increase in total cholesterol (Tohen, Ketter et al., 2003). These issues can be addressed through careful management, such as monitoring blood levels and side effects, avoiding this option in patients with contraindicated health issues (i.e., obesity), and ongoing discussion of emerging concerns with patients during treatment.

Risperidone—Risperidone is indicated for treatment of manic and mixed symptoms. The efficacy of monotherapy risperidone in the treatment of manic and mixed symptoms has been supported by placebo-controlled trials (Hirschfeld, Keck et al., 2004; Khanna et al., 2005; Smulevich et al., 2005) and positive comparisons with other effective compounds (Perlis et al., 2006; Segal, Berk, & Brook, 1998; Smulevich et al., 2005). Risperidone is also available in an injectable, slow-absorbing intramuscular form, which is indicated for maintenance treatment (Quiroz et al., 2010; MacFadden et al., 2009).

Quetiapine—Quetiapine is effective for euphoric hypomanic or manic symptoms (Bowden et al., 2005; McIntyre et al., 2005a). For those patients who do not respond to monotherapy, quetiapine in combination with lithium or divalproex is also indicated for the treatment of acute mania (Sachs et al., 2004; Yatham, Paulsson, Mullen, & Vagero, 2004). Quetiapine is also offered in an extended release version, which has an additional indication for the acute treatment of mixed episodes.

Ziprasidone—Two double-blind, placebo-controlled trials in acute mania support the efficacy of ziprasidone for treatment of manic and mixed symptoms in bipolar disorder (Keck, Versiani et al., 2003; Potkin et al., 2005).

Special Considerations for Using Second-Generation Antipsychotic Medications Increased risk for obesity and type 2 diabetes, which can be exacerbated by weight gain observed in varying degrees in members of this class of medications, suggests that monitoring of body weight, calculation of body mass index (BMI), and education about sound diet, nutrition, and exercise are important treatment components (Citrome & Jaffe, 2003).

At the 2004 Consensus Development Conference on Antipsychotic Drugs and Obesity and Diabetes, experts from the American Diabetes Association, American Psychiatric Association, American Association of Clinical Endocrinologists, and the North American Association for the Study of Obesity proposed a monitoring protocol for patients taking second-generation antipsychotic medications. Table 3.2 illustrates the protocol (ADA, APA, AACE, & NAASO, 2004).

Research is underway to determine whether second-generation antipsychotic medications have a direct effect on metabolism separate from secondary effects due to weight gain.

Using Combination Medications

Typically, published algorithms for treatment of bipolar disorder have recommended trying a single medication first, and then, if needed, combining medications (VA, DoD, 2010; Hirschfeld et al., 2002; Keck, Perlis, & Otto, 2004; Suppes, Dennehy et al., 2005; Yatham et al., 2009). The majority of patients with bipolar disorder will need more than one medication to achieve lasting mood stability. Recent studies suggest that the use of two medications to treat acute mania may increase the degree of response for many patients in the first three weeks of treatment (Sachs et al., 2004; Yatham et al., 2004; Tohen et al., 2002).

Combination therapy typically includes selections of medications from different drug classes, most notably combinations of lithium, anticonvulsants, and second-generation antipsychotic medications.

Table 3.2   Monitoring Protocol for Patients Taking Second-Generation Antipsychotics*

Screening Measures	Baseline	4 Weeks	8 Weeks	12 Weeks	Quarterly	Annually	Every 5 Years
Personal/family history	X					X	
Weight (BMI)	X	X	X	X	X		
Waist circumference	X			X		X	
Blood pressure	X			X		X	
Fasting plasma glucose	X			X		X	
Fasting lipid profile	X			X			X

*More frequent assessments may be warranted based on clinical status (ADA, APA, AACE, & NAASO, 2004).

Source: American Diabetes Association, American Psychiatric Association, American Association of Clinical Endocrinologists, North American Association for the Study of Obesity. (2004). Consensus development conference on antipsychotic drugs and obesity and diabetes. *Diabetes Care, 27*(2), 596–601.

What Medications Are Used to Treat Depression in Patients with Bipolar Disorder?

Figure 3.3 summarizes medications used to treat acute bipolar depression, including recommended dosages and side effects.

Medications used to treat depression in patients with bipolar disorder typically include lithium, valproate, and the second-generation antipsychotic medications as well as lamotrigine and antidepressants. The following section focuses exclusively on medications with evidence for support of their use in treatment of depressive symptoms in bipolar disorder.

Lithium—While not used with the frequency of other agents, lithium monotherapy is effective in treating depressive symptoms in patients with bipolar disorder. Lithium may also have unique protective effects in that it has been associated with decreased risk for suicidality (Baldessarini & Tondo, 2008; Baldessarini, Tondo, & Hennen, 2003; Ernst & Goldberg, 2004).

Valproate—There is a small but encouraging literature suggesting that valproate may be helpful in treatment of acute episodes of depression in bipolar disorder. Given the strength of its antimanic properties, inclusion of valproate in an overall treatment regimen may have multiple benefits.

Pramipexole—There have been two small, positive, double-blind, placebo-controlled studies of adjunctive pramipexole, a dopamine agonist used in the treatment of Parkinson's disease, in the treatment of bipolar I and bipolar II depression (Goldberg, Burdick, & Endick, 2004; Zarate Jr. et al., 2004).

Lamotrigine—The anticonvulsant lamotrigine has some acute antidepressant efficacy, but it is particularly effective in the prevention of new depressive episodes (see section on maintenance treatment options). The drug has a rare, potential side effect of medically serious rashes (Stevens Johnson syndrome or toxic epidermal necrolysis). This risk

absolute starting dose—amount of medication given when the patient first takes it

rate of initial titration—the rate by which a medication is increased to what is believed to be a minimum effective dose

is strongly associated with *absolute starting dose* and/or *rate of initial titration*. Thus, following the recommended dosing schedule is critical.

Second-Generation Antipsychotic Medications

Quetiapine—The finding that the second-generation antipsychotic medication quetiapine was helpful for bipolar depression was a significant advancement in treatment options for patients with bipolar depression. Quetiapine is approved for treatment of depressive episodes in both BDI and BDII, and is also available in an extended release formulation.

Olanzapine and Fluoxetine combination—The FDA-approved combination of olanzapine-fluoxetine HCL for

Figure 3.3 Medication Dosages and Common Side Effects for Treating Acute Phase Depression in Patients with Bipolar Disorder*

Type/Class: Medication	Usual Target Dose**	Usual Maximum Recommended Dose (level)	Recommended Administration Schedule	Common Side Effects***
Lithium (also available in a slow-absorption formula)	0.6-1.0 mEq/L	1.2 mEq/L	2 times daily or at bedtime	Tremor, drowsiness, nausea/vomiting, increased urine output, muscle weakness, thirst, dry mouth, cognitive impairment
Valproate	80 µg/mL	125 ug/mL	2 times daily or at bedtime	Nausea/vomiting, increased appetite with weight gain, sedation, hair loss, reversible increases in liver function tests, reversible thrombocytopenia, rarely pancreatitis
Lamotrigine	200	600 mg/day	Once daily	Headache, nausea, rash, dizziness, ataxia, somnolence, rhinitus
Pramipexole	1–3 mg/day	4.5 mg/day	3 times daily	Nausea, dizziness, constipation, hallucinations, insomnia, muscle weakness, confusion, and abnormal movements
SSRIs Citalopram	20–40	60 mg/day	Once daily	Dizziness, dry mouth, insomnia, agitation, nausea, sexual dysfunction, headache
Escitalopram	10–20	20 mg/day	Once daily	
Fluoxetine	20	80 mg/day	Once daily	
Fluvoxamine	150–250	250 mg/day	Once daily	
Paroxetine	20–50	60 mg/day	Once daily	
Sertraline	100	290 mg/day	Once daily	
Other Antidepressants Bupropion	300	450 mg/day	2–3 times daily	Headache, agitation, weight loss, insomnia, nausea, seizure, dry mouth, dizziness
Trazodone	300–600	600 mg/day	Once daily	Drowsiness, dizziness, headache, blurred vision, sedation, orthostatic hypotension, dry mouth, constipation
Venlafaxine	150	375 mg/day	Once daily	Dizziness, somnolence, insomnia, decreased appetite, anxiety, headache, nausea, sexual dysfunction, potential elevation in blood pressure at higher doses

(continued)

Figure 3.3   *(Continued)*

Duloxetine	40–60 mg/day	60 mg/day	Once daily	Nausea, dry mouth, constipation, somnolence, hyperhidrosis, decreased appetite
Second-Generation Antipsychotics: Olanzapine and Fluoxetine	6–25	12–50 mg/day	At bedtime	See side effects noted for SSRIs (above) and olanzapine, quetiapine (Figure 3.1)
Quetiapine	300–600	800 mg/day	At bedtime Once daily	

*This review of medications is intended to provide information on commonly used medications, but not to be comprehensive. Additionally, this information is not intended to provide prescription information, and a physician or appropriate individual should be consulted prior to making medication changes. For full information about medications, physicians should carefully review package inserts for individual medications or access the Physicians' Desk Reference.
**Doses used for maintenance treatment may be lower.
***Side effects may be less with slow-absorbing forms of medications. Lithium, divalproex, carbamazepine, and quetiapine are available in slow-absorption (or extended-release) formulations.

> There is growing support for the use of the second-generation antipsychotic medications quetiapine and olanzapine (administered in combination with fluoxetine) for the treatment of bipolar depression. Use of these medications must be weighed against consideration of side effects and safety considerations.

treatment of bipolar depression provides three dose formulations. Because olanzapine is a recognized antimanic agent, using this combination requires no additional antimanic medication unless indicated by individual patient needs.

For both of these medications, positive efficacy trials must be balanced against concern about weight gain and development of hyperlipidemia, hyperglycemia, or diabetes. Safety and monitoring considerations mentioned previously (page 41) also apply for the use of second-generation antipsychotics in the treatment of bipolar depression.

Antidepressant Medications

Importantly, most of the evidence in support of these medications comes from studies in unipolar depression. Despite a lack of strong evidence in support of their use, antidepressant medications are commonly prescribed for treatment of bipolar depression. While medications from the selective serotonin reuptake inhibitor class (SSRI) are most commonly used, clinicians may choose from a wide variety of available antidepressant medications with some demonstrated efficacy in the treatment of depression.

Antidepressants are generally started following remission of manic symptoms if depression develops or if a patient was euthymic (not manic or depressed) and develops new depressive symptoms. If a person is experiencing mood instability or rapid cycling, use of antidepressants may actually worsen or prolong the period of instability.

If used, there are little data to distinguish the effectiveness of using one type of antidepressant over another, so virtually all antidepressants are used in bipolar disorder treatment (Post et al., 2006). Importantly, patients need to be aware that all medications used to treat depression will require two to three weeks to see an improvement of symptoms. Often close family members or friends will notice improvement before the patient does.

Antidepressants typically used for treating patients with bipolar disorder include the following:

> **SSRI medications,** which enhance serotonergic transmission, are in widespread clinical use. These are administered as a single, daily dose, which may potentially increase compliance.

> **Bupropion** has little side-effect impact on sexual functioning, relatively few drug interactions, and reasonable tolerability.

> **Trazodone** is sometimes used in low doses to help with sleep problems associated with depressive symptoms.

> **Venlafaxine** and **duloxetine** are antidepressants that enhance both noradrenergic and serotonergic neurotransmitters, usually administered twice daily.

Effectiveness of Medications for Treating Depression in Bipolar Disorder

There are remarkably few data on treatment of depression in bipolar disorder, and most treatment recommendations are based on expert consensus and common clinical practice rather than scientifically rigorous studies. A striking contrast is the recent work done on the effectiveness of the second-generation antipsychotics quetiapine (monotherapy) and olanzapine (in combination with the SSRI medication fluoxetine) in the treatment of bipolar depression. However, as with all medication choices, a balance of efficacy and tolerability must be considered. There are tremendous individual differences in response and sensitivity to side effects in all medications discussed.

Lithium

A number of studies conclude that lithium may be effective for treatment of depression in persons with bipolar disorder (Bauer & Dopfmer, 1999; Ebert, Jaspert, Murata, & Kaschka, 1995; Fieve, Kumbaraci, & Dunner, 1976; Post et al., 1997; Prien, Caffey, & Klett, 1973). However, lithium is most often used in combination with another agent for the treatment of acute depressive episodes in bipolar disorder. A recent trial demonstrated that for patients not fully responsive to lithium monotherapy for acute depression, the addition of lamotrigine was significantly better than placebo (van der Loos et al., 2009).

Continuing controversy exists as to the long-term use of antidepressants with mood stabilizers in those with bipolar I disorder (Belmaker, 2007). Side-effect profile and clinical response varies among antidepressants; multiple trials may be necessary to find the best medication for a given individual.

Antidepressant discontinuation should be done gradually unless there is a medical need to stop abruptly, such as intolerable side effects.

Because medication responsiveness and side effects differ from one individual to another, and because of the increasing treatment options and combinations available, it is important to work closely with each patient to optimize medications.

Valproate

There are two small ($n = 25$ and 18) positive placebo-controlled double-blind studies of divalproex in patients with bipolar depression (Davis et al., 2005; Ghaemi et al., 2007). While these are encouraging preliminary findings, larger controlled trials are necessary to establish the role of valproate in the treatment of acute depressive episodes in bipolar disorder.

Pramipexole

Two small positive placebo-controlled studies for pramipexole, a dopamine agonist, suggest that it may be a helpful alternative for those who don't respond to more conventional therapies. In the first study (Goldberg et al., 2004), 22 patients with treatment-resistant BDI and BDII were randomized to pramipexole ($n = 12$; mean dose = 1.7 mg/day) or placebo ($n = 10$) for 6 weeks. In the second study (Zarate Jr. et al., 2004), 21 inpatients and outpatients with BDII were randomized to pramipexole ($n = 10$; mean dose = 1.7 mg/day) or placebo ($n = 11$) for 6 weeks. Both studies showed significant benefit compared to placebo, and there was no significant risk of switching into hypomania or mania during short-term treatment.

Lamotrigine

Although multiple placebo-controlled monotherapy trials of lamotrigine for depressive episodes in bipolar disorder failed to show significant efficacy individually, a pooled analysis suggested some benefit (Calabrese et al. 2008; Geddes, Calabrese, & Goodwin, 2009), particularly for more severely depressed patients. A placebo-controlled comparison to the combination of olanzapine and fluoxetine ("OFC") likewise suggested some benefit (Brown et al., 2006). While OFC was superior in efficacy, lamotrigine has a more benign side effect profile. A recent study has also demonstrated the effectiveness of lamotrigine in combination with lithium (van der Loos et al., 2009).

Lamotrigine has a rare, potential side effect of medically serious rashes (Stevens Johnson syndrome or toxic epidermal necrolysis). This risk is strongly associated with *absolute starting dose* and/or *rate of initial titration*. Thus, following the recommended medication-dosing schedule is critical.

Second-Generation Antipsychotics

Quetiapine—In recent years, the benefit of quetiapine monotherapy for the acute treatment of bipolar depression has been demonstrated in four large, multicenter, placebo-controlled trials. Importantly, all four trials included participants with bipolar I and II disorder, and also allowed those with rapid cycling. These included two identical

8-week placebo-controlled studies enrolling more than 1000 patients combined (Calabrese et al., 2005a; Thase et al., 2006), and 8-week placebo-controlled comparisons to paroxetine (McElroy et al., 2010) and lithium (Young, Carlsson, Olausson, Paulsson, & Brecher, 2008). Similar findings were observed in an 8-week placebo controlled trial of extended release quetiapine (Suppes et al., 2010).

Olanzapine-Fluoxetine Combination ("OFC")—A recent placebo-controlled study in depressed patients with BDI found significant efficacy for the combination of olanzapine (a second-generation antipsychotic) and fluoxetine (an SSRI) without an increased risk for development of mania (Tohen, Vieta et al., 2003). In this study, the use of olanzapine alone was also significant relative to placebo, although the results were not as striking nor of the same effect size as the combination.

For more information on special considerations for using second-generation antipsychotics, see pages 40–41.

SSRIs and Other Antidepressants

Despite the broad use of antidepressants for treatment of depression in bipolar disorder, there are limited controlled trials assessing their effectiveness (Boerlin et al., 1998; Gijsman et al., 2004; Kupfer et al., 2001; Vieta et al., 2002). A recent large randomized trial ($n = 366$) assessed the benefit of adding antidepressant medications (paroxetine or bupropion) or placebo to mood-stabilizing medications in patients with bipolar I or bipolar II disorder in a depressive episode (Sachs et al., 2007). Antidepressants were not associated with increased effectiveness in this trial. Quetiapine was superior to paroxetine in an 8-week randomized controlled trial of acute depression in bipolar disorder (McElroy et al., 2008). Clinicians have been educated to use caution when prescribing antidepressants in this population due to concerns about the risk of inducing a "switch" into mania (Leverich et al., 2006; Post et al., 2006). However, this risk is fairly low (about 5-12 percent) compared to placebo when antidepressants are added to effective antimanic medications (Post et al., 2001, 2006).

For patients with particularly treatment-resistant depressive symptoms, clinicians may consider using antidepressant drugs from the mono-amine oxidase inhibitors (MAOIs) or tricyclic class of drugs. These choices are associated with more safety concerns and monitoring requirements. These medications have demonstrated effectiveness for treatment of major depressive episodes in a number of smaller studies (Cohn, Collins, Ashbrook, & Wernicke, 1989; Himmelhoch, Thase, Mallinger, & Houck, 1991; Ketter, Post, Parekh, & Worthington, 1995; Nemeroff et al., 2001; Sachs et al., 1994; Thase, Mallinger, McKnight, & Himmelhoch, 1992).

What Strategies Are Recommended for Maintenance Treatment?

There are relatively few scientific studies on the long-term management of patients with bipolar disorder. In practice, virtually all patients need ongoing antimanic medication to prevent symptom relapse; however, the overall medication burden often can be minimized during maintenance treatment. For those taking a combination of mood stabilizers, the clinician should taper one medication associated with either side effects or partial response, while continuing other medications. Current general practice guidelines for those with BDI support lifetime treatment following two manic episodes, or following one episode if severe and/or a significant family history of bipolar or major depressive disorder exists. While ongoing treatment is generally recommended, at minimum, those with BDII should maintain contact with a clinician and participate in treatment as necessary.

For those patients who are prescribed an antidepressant medication, usual maintenance recommendations are to gradually taper antidepressant treatment following symptom remission and after a period of stability lasting at least two to four months. However, some patients with bipolar disorder may need continuous antidepressant treatment along with antimanic agents (Altshuler et al., 2003). As early as the 1970s, researchers noticed that antimanic medications sometimes pushed the brain below a euthymic level, thus necessitating use of antidepressants to balance the brain chemistry.

Maintenance treatment should involve the fewest possible medications at the lowest possible dose that will achieve ongoing mood stabilization.

Clinicians and patients need to carefully collaborate on the initiation and duration of maintenance pharmacological management. Key issues to resolve are:

- ► Personal preference and response
- ► Risk factors for recurrence
- ► Side-effect profile
- ► Ability to tolerate the prescribed medication (critical to ensuring long-term adherence to maintenance therapy)
- ► Concomitant medical concerns or other psychiatric diagnoses.

Effectiveness of Maintenance Treatment for Bipolar Patients

The goal of maintenance treatment is to prolong periods of stability by preventing new mood episodes. The following medications have FDA indications in support of their use as maintenance therapy in bipolar disorders: lithium, lamotrigine, aripiprazole, olanzapine, risperidone IM, quetiapine and quetiapine XR, and ziprasidone. Some of them have evidence in support of their use as monotherapy, while others are effective in combination with lithium or valproate. It is usually preferable to continue therapy with the agent that contributed to initial stabilization during the acute phase rather than switch to something different in maintenance phase treatment. Importantly, selection of medications for maintenance therapy involves long-term use, and clinicians and patients must carefully weigh any associated side effects as well as efficacy in prevention of new mood episodes.

Lithium

A meta-analysis of the five most rigorously designed studies of maintenance treatment with lithium concluded that lithium significantly reduced the overall risk of mood episodes (relative risk = 0.66) and manic episodes (relative risk = 0.62), but not depressive episodes (Geddes, Burgess, Hawton, Jamison, & Goodwin, 2004). In a pooled analysis of 18-month studies of lithium compared to lamotrigine, lithium was more effective than lamotrigine in prevention of manic episodes ($p = 0.03$; Goodwin et al., 2004). The suggestion that lithium may have a protective effect of reducing the risk of self-harm may also support its selection as a maintenance treatment.

Anticonvulsants

Lamotrigine—For those who tolerate and respond to lamotrigine monotherapy in acute treatment, it is an important option in maintenance treatment due to its effectiveness in decreasing the likelihood of new depressive episodes (Bowden et al., 2003; Calabrese et al., 2003). Lamotrigine was compared to lithium in two large, 18-month, randomized, double-blind, placebo-controlled studies. One study enrolled patients who were recently manic or hypomanic ($n = 175$), while the other enrolled those who were recently depressed ($n = 463$) (Bowden et al., 2003; Calabrese et al., 2003). The data from the two studies were then combined in a pooled analysis (Goodwin et al., 2004). In both trials, patients who improved during the open-treatment phase with lamotrigine were randomly assigned to maintenance treatment with lamotrigine, lithium, or placebo; thus the study population was "enriched" with those who benefit from lamotrigine in acute phase treatment. For the primary outcome measure (time until additional pharmacotherapy was required for treatment of a mood episode), lamotrigine was superior to placebo ($p < 0.001$). Lamotrigine showed benefit in preventing both manic ($p = 0.034$) and depressive episodes ($p = 0.009$), although the magnitude of benefit was greater for prevention of depression.

Valproate—The long-term effectiveness of divalproex compared to lithium and placebo was studied in one large ($n = 372$) placebo-controlled, double-blind, randomized trial

(Bowden et al., 2000). In this study, there was no significant difference in the primary efficacy measure (time until development of any mood episode) between divalproex and placebo, although divalproex was superior to placebo on some secondary outcome measures such as rate of early termination for any mood episode (24 percent versus 38 percent, respectively; p <0.02) and early termination for depression (6 percent versus 16 percent; p <0.02). A reanalysis of this study examining only the subset of patients who were stabilized with divalproex prior to randomization found that these patients had significantly fewer recurrences when randomized to continue divalproex rather than change to placebo or lithium (McElroy et al., 2008). Another controlled, double-blind study (n = 251) comparing divalproex to olanzapine demonstrated equivalent effectiveness in prevention of new mood episodes (Tohen et al., 2003).

Carbamazepine—Although there is no formal FDA indication for the use of carbamazepine in maintenance treatment, an open-label study found that an extended-release formulation of carbamazepine was effective for those recently experiencing manic/mixed symptoms (Ketter, Kalali, & Weisler, 2004).

Second-Generation Antipsychotics

Many of the newer second-generation antipsychotic medications have some indications for maintenance therapy in bipolar disorder. Olanzapine and aripiprazole are both indicated as monotherapy maintenance treatments in bipolar disorder (Keck et al., 2006, 2007; Tohen et al., 2003, 2005, 2006). They may be more effective at delaying time to manic or hypomanic relapse as compared to depression. Risperidone IM is approved as a maintenance therapy, as monotherapy, or in combination with lithium or valproate (Quiroz et al., 2010; MacFadden et al., 2009).

Ziprasidone, quetiapine, and quetiapine XR are recommended maintenance treatments in combination with either lithium or valproate, based on large placebo-controlled trials (Bowden et al., 2010; Suppes et al., 2009; Vieta et al., 2008b).

Clozapine has proven to have some effectiveness for maintenance treatment in recent studies. It is recommended for treatment-resistant patients but requires ongoing monitoring for adverse events (ADA et al., 2004; Ketter et al., 2004; Suppes et al., 1999).

Antidepressants

For antidepressants, no definitive research exists to resolve questions regarding use in maintenance treatment. On one hand, many published treatment guidelines recommend stopping antidepressants within a few weeks or months after resolution of depressive symptoms. However, a retrospective study suggests that those patients who continue to take an antidepressant in combination with an antimanic medication for one year following a depressive episode have fewer clinical symptoms, function better, and are not at increased risk for switch into mania (Altshuler et al., 2003). These important data need to be addressed in a randomized prospective study to clarify recommendations for the long-term management of patients with chronic and severe depressive symptoms.

How Can Medication Treatment of Side Effects Be Managed?

Key side effects that patients with bipolar disorder may experience with medication therapy include gastrointestinal upset, tremor, sedation, extrapyramidal symptoms (Parkinson-like side effects, such as flat facial expression, stiff muscles, and slowed movements), *tardive dyskinesia*, insomnia, and sexual dysfunction.

A key clinical treatment issue in managing patients' medications is **how** changes are made. Always overlap a new medication with ongoing medications, and gradually taper any medication being discontinued unless there is a medical necessity to rapidly stop (e.g., allergic reaction or severe side effects). For full information about medications, physicians should carefully review package inserts for individual medications or access the *Physicians' Desk Reference* as well as other pertinent source documents.

Another critical aspect of managing side effects is monitoring for potential drug interactions. Drugs taken for heart, renal, endocrinologic, or hepatic disease may interact with lithium or other antimanic/antidepressive medications. Patients should be questioned about over-the-counter medication use as well.

How Are Electroconvulsive Therapy (ECT) and Alternative Medicine Used to Treat Patients with Bipolar Disorder?

ECT is an effective treatment for acute mania as well as for depression, whether in patients with bipolar or unipolar disorder (Mukherjee, Sackeim, & Schnurr, 1994; Small et al., 1988). However, safety, tolerability, and patient acceptance issues typically rank ECT behind pharmacological approaches. Due to the range of medications now available, ECT is reserved for patients unresponsive to or unable to take current medications, women who are pregnant, and patients in acute danger of committing

Clinicians need to carefully discuss both response and side effects with patients, emphasizing that, for the vast majority of patients, bipolar disorder requires lifelong treatment.

tardive dyskinesia— development of involuntary motor movements, which may persist beyond use of the medication, usually associated with first-generation antipsychotics

*Figure 3.4 presents a summary of recommendations compiled from the **Physicians' Desk Reference** for these side effects. This list is neither comprehensive nor intended to replace medical evaluation of side effects, but provides a general example of some of the most utilized approaches to management of side effects in this population.*

Figure 3.4   Treating Bipolar Disorder Medication Side Effects

Side Effects	Recommendations
GI Upset	• Administer medication with food and large quantities of liquid. • Consider lowering dose, if possible. • Use sustained-release preparations of medications when available. • Some data suggest that this side effect can be successfully treated with H2 blockers (e.g., cimetidine, ranitidine).
Tremor	**Enhanced physiologic tremor—A fine tremor of approximately 8–10 Hz; made worse when hands are outstretched** • Check blood levels of medication. • Decrease dose, divide dose, or change to slow-absorption preparation of the medication. • Propranolol can be given at 20–30 mg, 3 times daily, or 80 mg long-acting, daily. **Parkinsonian tremor—Coarse tremor at rest of approximately 4–6 Hz.** • Decrease dose, divide dose, use bedtime dosing, or switch to alternate medication. • Pharmacological treatments include benztropine 1–2 mg twice daily, amantadine 100 mg, 2 or 3 times daily, and diphenhydramine 25–50 mg, 2 or 3 times daily.
Sedation	• Change to bedtime dosing. • Substitute a less sedating, alternative medication.
Extrapyramidal Symptoms (EPS)	• Treat tremor as suggested above. • Reduce dose of antipsychotic medication. • Akathisia may respond to propranolol 20–30 mg, 3 times a day (or 80 mg slow-absorbing form, daily), benztropine, amantadine, or diphenhydramine. If ineffective, alternatives include clonidine (0.1 mg, 3 times a day) and lorazepam (1–2 mg, 2–3 times daily). • Dystonic reactions can often be prevented by benztropine 1 mg 2 or 3 times daily for the first few days of antipsychotic therapy. Acute dystonic reactions are generally managed with benztropine 1–2 mg or lorazepam 1 mg intramuscular.
Tardive Dyskinesia (TD)	• Prescribe antipsychotics in the lowest dose necessary for the shortest time possible. • Consider alternatives for mood stabilization and control of agitation. • Use second-generation antipsychotic medications, which appear to have a lower incidence of TD. Clozapine has also been helpful to minimize symptoms of TD. • Some evidence that vitamin E given in high doses (> 1000 units per day) may decrease some symptoms of TD for some patients.
Insomnia	• Use morning dosing, or spread total daily dose as early in the day as possible. • Use QHS dosing for any potentially sedating medications. • Use zolpidem (5–10 mg), zaleplon (5–20 mg; 10 mg recommended dose), or eszopiclone (1–3 mg) at bedtime, or a benzodiazepine, such as temazepam (15–30 mg), at night. Antipsychotics should always be considered second- or third-line agents for insomnia due to the risk of extrapyramidal symptoms, tardive dyskinesia, and other side effects. Avoid use of higher doses of trazodone for sleep as it is an antidepressant and thus has the potential for destabilizing and increasing symptoms of mania in patients with bipolar disorder. Benzodiazepines are best avoided in patients with prior history of substance abuse/dependence or who are at risk for substance abuse. Nonaddicting agents are preferred.
Sexual Dysfunction	• Add yohimbine at 4–7.5 mg, 3 times a day, cyproheptadine at 4–8 mg given shortly before sexual intercourse, or the antidepressant bupropion given at dosages of 75–300 mg per day. Bupropion has the advantage of potentially also augmenting the antidepressant efficacy of the SSRI.

suicide or who suffer dangerous lack of food and fluid intake due to severe depressive symptoms. The response to this treatment is quite rapid, with striking improvements seen often within one to two weeks.

In addition to ECT, other techniques such as repetitive transcranial magnetic stimulation (rTMS) and *vagal nerve stimulation* are now being explored. In rTMS, a pulsed magnetic field stimulates electrical activity in the brain. The magnetic field is generated by passing brief current pulses through a coil of wire, which is held close to the scalp to target certain brain areas. In vagal nerve stimulation, a pacemaker is inserted and a wire wrapped around the vagus nerve in the neck, which is then stimulated by a small electrical current every few minutes. The mechanism of efficacy of these procedures is unknown. Although most of the studies of these newer approaches involve only a small proportion of patients with bipolar depression, a 1-year open study of VNS in 9 patients with treatment-resistant rapid cycling bipolar disorder did suggest some benefit (Marangell et al., 2008).

vagal nerve stimulation— an FDA-approved treatment for refractory epilepsy and depression now being explored for bipolar disorder

There is growing interest in other alternative therapies including adjunctive treatments using fish oils (omega-3), acupuncture, and mineral supplements. Despite great interest, the evidence in support of the omega-3 fatty acids in mood stabilization remains mixed, although adjunctive therapy can be beneficial for other health reasons (Marangell et al., 2006). Recent small studies assessing the benefit of acupuncture for symptoms of both hypomania and depression in bipolar disorder suggested that it was possible to target the symptom of interest with acupuncture stimulation, although acupuncture treatment did not separate from control conditions, which may have been active treatments themselves (Dennehy et al., 2009).

Caution should be exercised before embracing alternative or complementary approaches. For example, kava kava (an herb sometimes used to combat anxiety) has been associated with cases of liver failure (Ernst, 2002). Clinicians should query patients about their use of alternative or complementary treatments at every visit.

How Does the Presence of Co-Occurring Disorders Impact Medication Treatment for Bipolar Disorder?

Bipolar disorder often co-occurs with other psychiatric illnesses, including:

▶ Alcohol and/or substance abuse or dependence

> ► Anxiety disorders (e.g., panic, general anxiety, obsessive-compulsive, and post-traumatic stress disorders)

> ► Impulse control disorders

For patients with these co-occurring illnesses, symptom resolution may be slower and may require careful selection of medications to address all symptoms while minimizing medication burden.

Key Concepts for Chapter 3

1. Identification of effective treatments for bipolar disorder has increased options for patients and clinicians.

2. Treatment of bipolar I disorder must include antimanic medications.

3. For hypomania/mania, classes of effective medications used include lithium, anticonvulsants, and second-generation antipsychotics; a balanced treatment approach must consider efficacy, tolerability, and safety data.

4. Combination treatment is recommended at the outset for treating more severe manic symptoms.

5. It is important to treat the depressive phase of the illness because of the potential for suicide and impact on quality of life. However, there are limited data to recommend the use of antidepressant medications, while data are accumulating in favor of quetiapine and the combination of olanzapine and fluoxetine.

6. Maintenance treatment is recommended for all patients diagnosed with bipolar I disorder. There is now more data to guide choice of maintenance-phase treatments.

7. Medications used to treat bipolar disorder often cause side effects, which must be minimized to maintain adherence to treatment.

8. There is growing interest in the use of alternative and complementary medicine to treat associated symptoms of bipolar disorder. More research is needed to explore these alternative options.

Chapter 4
Psychosocial Treatments for Bipolar Disorder

This chapter answers the following questions:

▶ **Why Add Psychosocial Interventions to Pharmacotherapy?**—This section discusses psychosocial therapy's adjunctive treatment role for improving medication adherence, coping with stress, preventing relapse, and improving functioning and quality of life.

▶ **What Psychosocial Interventions Are Used to Treat Bipolar Disorder?**—This section presents an overview of the types of successful interventions used as adjunct therapy to medication.

▶ **What Is the Psychoeducational Approach to Bipolar Disorder Treatment?**—This section covers key elements of psychoeducational treatment strategies and the effectiveness of psychoeducation.

▶ **What Is Family-Focused Treatment (FFT) for Bipolar Disorder?**—This section covers FFT (psychoeducation, communication awareness, and problem-solving skills) as well as results of recent efficacy studies.

▶ **What Individual Psychosocial Approaches Are Used to Treat Bipolar Disorder?**—This section reviews cognitive-behavioral therapy (CBT) and interpersonal social rhythm therapy (IPSRT). Results of efficacy studies follow each treatment discussion.

▶ **Which Psychosocial Approaches Are Best for the Treatment of Bipolar Disorder?**—This study reviews comparative studies of different treatment approaches.

P SYCHOSOCIAL treatments for bipolar disorder have evolved over the years. Initially, psychosocial therapy was the only clinical option for treatment of bipolar disorder. As effective medication treatments became available, interest in developing psychosocial treatments and research into the efficacy of these interventions waned. Although there is increased recognition that bipolar disorder is a "brain disease" requiring pharmacological treatment, it has become clear that psychosocial therapies are important and useful adjuncts to medication, and can also positively impact brain function. Today, psychosocial interventions, including *psychoeducation* and more traditional therapies, once again play an important role in treating bipolar disorder.

Knowledge about the effectiveness of psychosocial interventions for different symptoms and phases of illness in bipolar disorder is increasing.

psychoeducation— teaching patients and/or family members about the illness, treatments, and relapse prevention

Why Add Psychosocial Interventions to Pharmacotherapy?

Both psychosocial therapy outcome studies and published treatment guidelines support the use of psychosocial treatment approaches as an adjunct to pharmacological therapy.

Recent reviews of psychosocial therapy outcome studies in bipolar disorder conclude that adjunctive psychoeducational and cognitive-behavioral strategies result in a decreased rate of hospitalization and incidence of relapse as well as improved medication adherence and overall clinical symptoms (Gonzalez-Pinto et al., 2004; Miklowitz, 2008; Otto et al., 2003; Swartz & Frank, 2001).

> *Psychosocial treatments for bipolar disorder tend to focus on the management of life circumstances that impact course of illness, as well as improving recognition and prevention of new episodes.*

Published guidelines for treating bipolar disorder also support the use of psychosocial interventions. For example, the Expert Consensus Guideline for bipolar disorder includes psychotherapy plus medication as one of the first options in treatment of depression in bipolar disorder (Keck et al., 2004). Evidence suggests that psychosocial therapy may improve adherence to treatment, teach better coping mechanisms to deal with stressful life events, teach tactics to prevent relapse, and improve overall functioning and quality of life.

Improving Adherence to Medication Treatment

Despite advances in effective medication treatments for bipolar disorder, some people's symptoms do not completely remit or disappear. Only about 50–60 percent of acutely ill patients respond to lithium or anticonvulsants alone, and many require combinations of drugs, as described in Chapter 3. As medication combinations become more complex, the likelihood of side effects (e.g., weight gain, nausea, cognitive "dullness") increases and patients' willingness to comply with prescribed regimens decreases. Research indicates that only about 40 percent of patients are fully adherent with prescribed medication (Colom et al., 2005a; Lingam & Scott, 2002). Key reasons for patients to lapse or totally stop taking their medication(s) include:

> *Discontinuing medications, particularly without physician supervision, carries the risk of relapse, diminished response to future treatments, and a more severe course of illness.*
>
> *Clinicians and patients should not "settle" for medication(s) with undesired side effects which could potentially be used to justify lack of adherence.*

- ▶ Not wanting to lose what are perceived as beneficial and satisfying symptoms (i.e., hypomania)
- ▶ Finding the negative side effects of some medications intolerable
- ▶ Mistakenly thinking that, by not experiencing an episode in some time, they have been "cured" and no longer require treatment

Optimum treatment of bipolar disorder occurs when psychosocial interventions augment pharmacological treatments. Several studies suggest that psychoeducation and interventions that address medication adherence significantly improve both adherence and clinical and functional outcomes. Because of these issues, psychosocial interventions for bipolar disorder emphasize education on the recurrent and lifelong nature of this illness and the importance of adherence to treatment regimens.

Coping with Stress

Psychosocial therapy can help patients deal with both the environmental and psychological factors that contribute to episode frequency and the rate of recovery from mood episodes. Evidence suggests that new episodes can be prompted by (Frank, Swartz, & Kupfer, 2000; Johnson & Roberts, 1995; Malkoff-Schwartz et al., 2000; Reilly-Harrington, Alloy, Fresco, & Whitehouse, 1999):

► Stressful life events

► Activities that disrupt the sleep/wake rhythms (working swing shifts or jet lag)

► Psychological factors, such as how one's attributional style and attitudes may interact with life events to predict increased symptoms

An example of an *attributional style* might be attributing negative life events (e.g., being laid off from a seasonal job) in terms of dispositional characteristics (e.g., "I was terrible on the cash register and made too many mistakes"). The person may experience more depressive symptoms than those who attribute the same event to external causes (e.g., "They don't need me anymore because the holiday rush is over").

attributional style—one's tendencies in making causal explanations about a variety of intra- and interpersonal events in one's life

People with chronic bipolar disorder may have limited social support, which can negatively impact their response to treatment. Absence of social support (e.g., having few friends) predicts a longer time to recovery after a manic, depressed, or mixed episode as well as higher levels of depression over six months (Johnson, Winett, Meyer, Greenhouse, & Miller, 1999).

Because of the connections between physical and environmental factors and course of illness, psychosocial interventions for patients with bipolar disorder might focus on:

► Increasing social support (e.g., working with the patient to improve existing relationships, or to establish and build new relationships)

► Teaching the importance of regulating sleep-wake cycles (e.g., working with the patient to establish a sleep "routine," such as going to bed by 11:00 p.m. each night and using an alarm clock to wake at a consistent hour)

► Teaching coping methods for stressful life events (e.g., assertive communication or relaxation techniques)

► Identifying and altering psychological mechanisms that exacerbate symptoms (e.g., a person's tendency to minimize symptoms and discontinue medications) and developing a strategy to correct that instinct

Preventing Relapse

Bipolar disorder is a lifetime condition characterized by re-
peated mood episodes. Despite previously adequate treatment,
individuals can experience relapse or the emergence of a new
mood episode (depression, hypomania, mania, or mixed) after
achieving remission. New research suggests that in addition to
medication, psychosocial interventions are helpful in the prevention of new episodes (Colom et al., 2003; Miklowitz et al., 2003;
Miklowitz et al., 2007). Individual or group interventions that emphasize psychoeducation, clinical management (i.e., adherence,
lifestyle changes, and early detection of *prodromal* symptoms),
interpersonal difficulties, or cognitive and behavioral factors are
associated with improved outcomes, including reduced risk of
recurrence and better functioning. The availability of effective
maintenance interventions is critical, because when patients experience longer intervals of wellness, their risk of a new episode
decreases (Tohen, Waternaux, & Tsuang, 1990).

prodromal—precursor to a
full episode, or less than criteria for a full-blown episode;
subsyndromal symptoms

Individuals need to learn to recognize external events that may
trigger an increase in symptoms (e.g., an upcoming family event
that has been stressful in the past). Additionally, psychosocial
treatment can help individuals learn to monitor themselves for
specific behaviors that are reliable warning signs of an increase
in symptoms or an emergent episode. These warning signs tend
to be unique for each individual, but once identified, they tend
to repeat and can be monitored and acted upon as a helpful relapse prevention tool. For example, a patient might identify restless sleep, increased irritability, and more frequent purchase of
lottery tickets as their key warning signs.

*Along with recognition of the
early warning signs, individuals
should have a plan for dealing
with them, including concrete
actions one can quickly take to
stabilize the situation, such as
calling the clinician.*

Finally, psychosocial treatment can help with relapse prevention
by facilitating the development of a plan to promote wellness,
such as regularly eating healthy meals, getting adequate sleep,
limiting or avoiding alcohol, and exercising.

Improving Functioning and Quality of Life

Even during periods of adequate medication treatment and relatively stable moods, many individuals with bipolar disorder continue to experience significant functional impairment (Bauer
et al., 2001; Judd et al., 2005; MacQueen et al., 2001).

At work, this ongoing dysfunction is evident in the finding that
six months after hospitalization, 30 percent of patients were unable to work at all, and only 21 percent worked at their expected
level (Dion, Tohen, Anthony, & Waternaux, 1988). At home, bipolar disorder is associated with high rates of family or marital

conflict, separation, and divorce (Coryell et al., 1993). Using psychosocial interventions to help develop coping skills for both manic and depressive symptoms may lessen the disorder's functional impact. Patients can learn to optimize their social and occupational functioning while coping with the diagnosis and treatment of a chronic illness.

> Even during periods of adequate medication treatment and relatively stable moods, many individuals with bipolar disorder continue to experience significant functional impairment (Bauer, Kirk, Gavin, & Williford, 2001; Judd et al., 2005; MacQueen et al., 2001).

What Psychosocial Interventions Are Used to Treat Bipolar Disorder?

Scott and Gutierrez (2004) present the commonalities among successful interventions. They include psychoeducation about bipolar disorder, encouragement of medication adherence, relapse prevention strategies, mood monitoring, and illness management skills. There is no clear "best" approach or combination for those with bipolar disorder (Miklowitz & Otto, 2006). Patients with symptoms of mood elevation may benefit more from interventions that focus on identification of emerging mood episodes and adherence to treatment, while those with primarily depressive symptoms may respond more to interventions that enhance cognitive and behavioral skills used to manage interpersonal relationships (Miklowitz, 2008).

Bauer and McBride (1996) describe key elements of psychosocial therapy of patients with bipolar disorder, summarized from descriptive reports of successful interventions. Figure 4.1 presents a brief overview of these elements and offers some overall guidance on what psychosocial interventions may be included in a treatment "package" for a patient with bipolar disorder.

From the Patient's Perspective

I'm really beginning to come to terms with what it means to have bipolar disorder. I don't think I really understood it in the beginning. It helps to have someone to talk with about having this illness, and to help me deal with some of the problems in my life. My husband is so angry with me for spending all the money, and I am trying to improve my communication skills so that he and I can get through this difficult time. I was also having such a hard time believing that this was something serious—I thought the doctor was just overreacting. But when I stopped my medication, I quickly figured out that these symptoms are serious, and they will come back if I don't take care of myself.

Figure 4.1   Elements of Successful Psychological Interventions for Bipolar Disorder

Type of Intervention	Elements of Intervention	Examples of Strategies within Element
Psychoeducational Interventions	• Education regarding illness and treatment	Informational videos or written materials about bipolar disorder
	• Illness management skills	Teaching strategies to remind patients to take medications as prescribed, such as alarms, pillboxes, or charts; rehearsal of steps to take when symptoms increase; education regarding the importance of treatment adherence
Problem-Solving/Coping Interventions	• Work management	Interventions to assist patient in navigating work problems, such as negotiating for a leave of absence
	• Family management	Interventions to assist patients coping with family issues, such as a relative who insists their problems are "all in their head"
	• Life goals outside of illness	Interventions to help patient reach life goals, such as completing school applications or starting a new hobby
Psychodynamic/Interpersonal Interventions	• Dealing with unstable interpersonal relationships	Interventions such as family or couples therapy to enhance relationship and communication with significant others
	• Coping with loss	Interventions that assist the patient to address and reduce feelings of grief and loss (may be loss due to death of a loved one, loss of plans and expectations set prior to illness, etc.)
	• Vulnerability	Interventions that assist the patient to develop resiliency and confidence
	• Self-concept	Interventions that assist the patient to develop a healthy and realistic sense of self

Source: Adapted from Bauer M, McBride L. *Structured Group Psychotherapy for Bipolar Disorder: The Life Goals Program.* New York: Springer Publishing Company, Inc., 1996.

Although research on psychosocial interventions for bipolar disorder is still limited, specific psychotherapies that have been shown to be effective for patients with bipolar disorder include the following:

- ▶ Psychoeducation
- ▶ Family-Focused Treatment (FFT)
- ▶ Individual treatments, such as Cognitive-Behavioral Therapy (CBT) and Interpersonal Social Rhythm Therapy (IPSRT)

What Is the Psychoeducational Approach to Bipolar Disorder Treatment?

Psychoeducation involves teaching patients and significant others, if available, about symptoms of bipolar disorder, treatment options, and prevention of relapse. Additionally, those close to the patient may learn coping strategies and problem-solving skills to help them deal more effectively with their loved one with bipolar disorder. Current thinking regarding the role of psychosocial treatments for bipolar disorder emphasizes an integrative approach, where one might pick and choose a different focus of education depending on illness and patient characteristics. For example, if a patient demonstrates a persistent problem taking medications as directed, psychoeducation for that person may focus on developing tools to help the person be more consistent (e.g., using a timer, pill box, or medication checklist posted in a prominent location in the home).

This section reviews the psychoeducational approach to treating bipolar disorder as well as findings from controlled research on its effectiveness when added to medication therapy.

Psychoeducational Treatment Strategies

Psychoeducational treatment strategies may focus on one or more of the following:

- ▶ **Taking prescribed medications as directed—** Helping the patient understand how medication adherence will improve symptoms and long-term course of illness, potentially prolonging periods of wellness between episodes, and reducing or minimizing mood symptoms when they do occur. Additionally, psychoeducation may include discussion of reasons people choose to discontinue medications and other treatments for bipolar disorder, and the possible consequences of that decision.

- ▶ **Understanding risk factors for relapse—**Patients will improve awareness of critical events or situations that make them more prone to relapse; for example, discontinuing medications, or experiencing particularly stressful life events, such as moving. With this knowledge and the awareness that these things may precipitate relapse, patients are more able to recognize and proactively respond if early symptoms emerge.

▶ **Recognizing warning signs of relapse**—Patients may learn to identify their own unique and individual warning signs that signal an emergent mood episode. For example, one individual may learn to recognize that sleeping greater than 10 hours per night usually occurs before the onset of a new depressive episode.

▶ **Managing stressful life events**—Helping the patient identify what life events can be particularly stressful and developing strategies (e.g., exercising, calling on supportive friends, or changing thought patterns) to better manage those events.

▶ **Protective factors**—Patients may learn to identify protective factors in their lives that support their treatment and management of bipolar symptoms (e.g., having daily contact with a family member or participating in a support group of friends).

It is critical to educate patients and their families about adherence to medication treatment, including the expected benefits of taking medications and what side effects they may experience.

Psychoeducation can be simple and straightforward (a patient and nurse discussing a new medication) or more complex and multifaceted (a structured psychoeducational curriculum administered in a group format). In psychoeducational interventions, patients learn to recognize signs and symptoms of their illness and take steps to prevent onset of new episodes. One helpful tool may be a daily Life Chart (Appendix C), which can be used by the individual to monitor and track daily moods and gain insight into how these relate to critical life events. As a psychoeducational tool (rather than a diagnostic tool as noted in Chapter 2), a Life Chart helps the patient learn to identify patterns in moods and to track the relationship of life events to mood changes. For example, a patient may realize that she regularly experiences increases in depressive symptoms at the time of her menses and can then strategize ways to anticipate and cope with these symptoms.

Appendix C includes a sample of a Life Chart.

Psychoeducation can be provided to groups of patients and/or families simultaneously (Colom et al. 2003; 2005b; Colom & Vieta 2006; Miller, Solomon, Ryan, & Keitner, 2004; Miller et al., 2008). Beyond beneficial effects associated with the supportive aspects of group participation, such interventions can target psychoeducational topics as well as issues pertaining to stigma, adaptation to living with a chronic illness, and problem-solving strategies.

Effectiveness of Psychoeducation

In many psychosocial interventions, psychoeducation is presented in the early phase of treatment and then other approaches are introduced as the patient's symptoms subside and treatment progresses (Bauer & McBride, 1996).

A recent, blind, controlled study of a structured psychoeducational intervention included 120 patients with BDI and BDII (Colom et al., 2003, 2005b). Outpatients in remission continued to receive standard pharmacologic treatment, and in addition, completed either 21 sessions of group psychoeducation or nonstructured group meetings led by a psychologist. Psychoeducation was significantly better than the control condition in preventing recurrence of any mood episode (60 vs. 38 percent; $p < .05$ in the 20-week treatment phase; 92 vs. 67 percent, $p < .001$ over a two-year follow-up period). Time to any recurrence was significantly longer for those in the psychoeducation group (log rank$_1$ = 13.45, $p < .001$). At the end of the 24-month follow-up period, number of days of hospitalization was significantly more for those in the control group (14.83 vs. 4.75 days for those in psychoeducation, $p < .05$). Additionally, serum lithium levels were higher and more stable in those receiving psychoeducation, indicating greater treatment adherence (Colom et al., 2005b).

Several large studies have evaluated interventions based on the Life Goals Program (Bauer & McBride, 1996), a structured group psychotherapy for bipolar disorder which includes a substantial psychoeducation component. The goals of this program are to improve illness management skills and social and occupational functioning. Bipolar patients ($n = 441$) were randomly assigned to pharmacotherapy alone or a care-management program consisting of pharmacotherapy plus structured group psychoeducation (Simon et al., 2005, 2006). Participation in the care management/psychoeducation component reduced the frequency and severity of mania in bipolar disorder; however, the effects were only observed among patients who entered with clinically significant mood symptoms.

In another large controlled evaluation of the Life Goals Program, Bauer et al. (2006a, b) randomized 330 bipolar patients from 11 VA sites around the United States to group-based psychoeducation combined with systematic chronic care management (CCM) or usual care. Group-based psychoeducation consisted of five weekly sessions led by a nurse, who also followed up with patients via twice-monthly contacts and continuity procedures based on the chronic care model (CCM). The sample was severely ill, and included individuals who had been recently hospitalized and had co-occurring substance use and medical disorders. Compared to usual VA care, psychoeducation and CCM significantly reduced weeks spent in an episode by 14

percent and weeks manic by 23 percent. While weeks spent depressed declined by 11 percent, this was not significant.
Significant improvements in social functioning, mental health–
related quality of life, and treatment satisfaction were also observed at different points during the 3-year follow-up period.

Family-focused therapy is the family treatment modality with the greatest amount of controlled research data in support of its use for adults and adolescents with bipolar disorder and their families. It combines elements of psychoeducation, family, cognitive, and behavioral therapies to address concerns most relevant to those with bipolar disorder.

What Is Family-Focused Treatment (FFT) for Bipolar Disorder?

FFT is a psychoeducational treatment approach that assumes
that the environmental setting within which a patient resides is
an important determinant of the likelihood of relapse. Therefore,
family psychoeducation is offered once a patient has begun to
stabilize from an acute episode. The program's goals are to educate patients and family members about the nature, symptoms,
course, and treatment of bipolar disorder. Additionally, a focus
on communication and problem-solving skills may reduce ten-
sion in the family environment.

FFT Treatment Strategies

FFT consists of 21 outpatient sessions held over nine months,
administered concurrently with ongoing pharmacotherapy. At
least one significant other (e.g., parent, spouse, sibling, supportive friend, caregiver) participates with the patient. Generally,
FFT includes three stages of treatment (Miklowitz & Goldstein,
1997):

1. **Family Psychoeducation**—In this stage, clinicians
   present educational materials on the illness, symptoms,
   risk and protective factors, origin of the disorder, medical
   and psychosocial treatments, importance of treatment
   adherence, and self-management tactics. Clinicians present the biological and genetic underpinnings of bipolar
   disorder from a vulnerability-stress perspective that emphasizes that, for a person who has a genetic propensity
   to the disorder, environmental stress can precipitate an
   episode and affect symptom severity. Additionally, this
   stage includes education about relapse prevention, in
   which participants learn to identify early warning signs
   and develop plans to prevent recurrence.

2. **Communication Enhancement Training**—In this
   stage, participants learn communication skills for dealing
   with family stress. These communication skills involve:
   - *Active listening*—This training teaches participants
     to listen attentively and incorporate verbal meaning,
     underlying feelings, emotions, and body language
     to their understanding of communication. Active

active listening—a way of listening that focuses entirely on what the other person is saying and confirms under-standing of both the message content and the emotions and feelings underlying the message to ensure accurate understanding

listening can include paraphrasing, or rephrasing someone's communication to ensure correct understanding. For example, the person may say, "I want to be sure I understand what you have said. You would like me to check with you before making purchases of more than $100. Is that correct?"

▶ **Expressing both positive and negative feelings**—Many people express their negative feelings, but neglect to mention those times when the behavior of another contributed to positive feelings. Communication enhancement training would emphasize relaying those messages, such as, "I felt very loved when you let me sleep late this morning."

▶ **Requesting adaptive changes in each other's behavior**—This training helps participants learn to request changes in family members, without using attacking or accusing language. For example, instead of saying, "You never help me around the house, and you just think I am lazy," a better way of requesting a change might be, "I've been feeling more depressed and have less energy right now. I'd like to split up some household chores so that they aren't as overwhelming to me during this hard time."

These critical communication and assertion skills are taught through *behavioral rehearsal* and *role-playing*.

3. **Problem-Solving Skills Training**—This final stage of FFT involves training participants to identify, define, and solve specific family problems related to bipolar disorder. For example, the family may be experiencing additional stress due to the patient having stopped working. This intervention may involve strategizing ways to cope with the reduced family income, staying within a budget, or discussing potential part- or full-time work options that may be feasible for the patient.

The FFT model includes between-session homework so that patients and family members can practice new skills at home. For example, they may be asked to use new *assertive communication techniques* in conversation and then report back on their success and problems implementing the techniques in real-life applications.

Effectiveness of FFT

A number of studies have been conducted in recent years on the efficacy of FFT as an adjunct to medication therapy compared to the following:

behavioral rehearsal—rehearsing new responses to problematic situations

role-playing—learning new communication skills by acting out conversations in therapeutic sessions

assertive communication techniques—these techniques help patients honestly express opinions, feelings, attitudes, and rights (without undue anxiety) in a way that doesn't infringe on the rights of others

FFT has been the subject of several controlled trials and is consequently the most well-known and validated family-based intervention for bipolar disorder.

▶ **Medication therapy alone**—FFT in addition to medication produced significantly less relapse (11 percent) than medication alone (61 percent) over a nine-month follow-up period (Miklowitz & Goldstein, 1997).

▶ **Two family education sessions and follow-up crisis management**—In the first randomized comparison of FFT compared to two family education sessions and follow-up crisis management (*n* = 70), 29 percent of patients who received FFT experienced a relapse into depression, compared to 53 percent in the comparison treatment, over a one-year follow-up period (Miklowitz et al., 2000). A larger trial (n = 101) indicated that patients receiving FFT experienced a 35 percent relapse rate, greater reduction in mood symptoms, and better medication adherence, compared to a 54 percent relapse rate, less reduction in mood symptoms, and poorer medication adherence for patients receiving 2 sessions of family education plus crisis intervention as needed (Miklowitz, George, Richards, Simoneau, & Suddath, 2003). Additionally, those in FFT averaged 73.5 weeks before a new mood episode versus 53.2 weeks for those in crisis management. Patients in both groups received concurrent medication treatment.

▶ **Individually focused treatment**—Patients participating in a nine-month study of FFT (concurrent with medication treatment) had only a 28 percent relapse rate in the year following the intervention period. Comparatively, patients in the control group receiving individual supportive, problem-focused, and educational interventions (concurrent with medication treatment) experienced a 60 percent relapse rate over the same follow-up period. Additionally, only 12 percent of patients in FFT were hospitalized during the posttreatment year, compared to 60 percent in individually based treatment (Rea et al., 2003).

A recent trial explored the use of FFT in 58 adolescents with bipolar disorders. Adolescents were randomized to receive either an adaptation of FFT (FFT-A) (Miklowitz, Biuckians, & Richards, 2006) and protocol pharmacotherapy (*n* = 30) or enhanced care (EC) and protocol pharmacotherapy (*n* = 28). Similar to adult FFT, FFT-A consisted of 21 sessions over 9 months with emphasis on psychoeducation, communication training, and problem-solving skills training. The EC consisted of three family sessions focused on relapse prevention. In comparison with adolescents treated with medication and three sessions of family psychoeducation (EC group), patients in FFT-A had shorter times to recovery from depression, less time in depressive episodes, and lower depression severity scores over the two-year treatment and observation period.

What Individual Psychosocial Therapy Approaches Are Used to Treat Bipolar Disorder?

This section presents treatment strategies and efficacy research results for cognitive behavioral therapy (CBT) and interpersonal social rhythm therapy (IPSRT).

CBT theory can be related to the philosophy of the ancient Greeks, "Nothing in life is actually bad, lest we perceive it to be so."

CBT Treatment Strategies

Cognitive-behavioral therapy (CBT) is most often associated with the work of Albert Ellis and Aaron Beck, dating back to the early 1970s. This therapy is based on the theory that dysfunctional or chronic, intense emotions stem from distorted and irrational thoughts. These thoughts are internalized by patients but impact their behaviors and patterns of social reinforcement. Thus, for CBT theorists, individuals' perceptions of life events can produce independent emotional and behavioral problems and potentially exacerbate symptoms of bipolar disorder and impact treatment response.

According to CBT, **"activating events"** (situational triggers) lead to **beliefs** (distorted and irrational thoughts), which lead to emotional and behavioral **consequences** (depression, anger, suicide attempts).

ACTIVATING EVENTS *(Situational Triggers)*

+

BELIEFS (*Distorted and Irrational Thoughts*)

=

CONSEQUENCES *(Depression, Anger,*

Suicide Attempts)

For example, being turned down for a date (an activating event) may trigger an individual to have irrational thoughts (beliefs), such as:

- ▶ "He hates me," rather than, "He said no to going on a date."
- ▶ "Nobody will ever like me," rather than, "Maybe I'm not his type."

> ▶ "I'll never find anybody who will love me," rather than, "The timing wasn't good for him; maybe he's involved with someone else."

> ▶ "That's it! Trying to make new relationships will never work. I'll have to be alone for the rest of my life," rather than, "Maybe next time, I'll find out more about the person as a friend, then I'll know more about whether to ask him out."

The results of these thought processes could be behaviors (consequences) such as withdrawing from social interaction, becoming depressed, or attempting suicide.

The cognitive-behavioral approach to the treatment of bipolar disorder is based on two underlying assumptions:

1. Thoughts, feelings, and behaviors are interrelated.
2. Patients who are well educated about their illness are better prepared to participate in their treatment and recovery.

Although many CBT-based theoretical interventions include some elements of psychoeducation, they also include cognitive restructuring and behavioral approaches, which differentiate them from a strictly psychoeducational approach to treatment.

CBT is an active therapy that involves ongoing interaction between clinician and patient. Most often, it involves mutually agreed-upon goals for change and continuously monitoring progress toward achieving those goals. For example, a patient and clinician may agree that minimizing irritable outbursts toward family members is a goal, and the patient will then keep a diary tracking unpleasant or hostile interactions with family members. It often includes homework assignments between sessions, such as completing relaxation exercises or practicing assertive communication skills. The goal of CBT is that patients will learn new skills and strategies that they will eventually implement independently.

Although CBT is commonly used for a multitude of psychological problems and psychiatric disorders, the focus for patients with bipolar disorder is somewhat more specific. As summarized in Basco and Rush (2005), goals of CBT for patients with bipolar disorder include teaching patients (and often significant others):

> ▶ About the disorder, treatment options, and common difficulties associated with the illness.

> ▶ Ways to monitor occurrence, severity, and course of manic and depressive symptoms and to change behaviors as needed (e.g., excessive daytime sleeping or gambling) and use structured problem solving as an alternative.

> ▶ Strategies for adhering to prescribed medication.

> ▶ How to use nonpharmacological strategies, specifically cognitive-behavioral skills, for coping with the cognitive,

affective, and behavioral problems associated with manic and depressive symptoms. For example, the goal may be to reduce dysfunctional cognitions and emotions associated with symptoms that lead to maladaptive behavior (e.g., thoughts of worthlessness leading to suicidal behavior).

▶ Coping strategies for stressors that may interfere with treatment or precipitate episodes of mania and/or depression.

Effectiveness of CBT

Several studies indicate that specific and targeted CBT is a helpful adjunct to pharmacotherapy for persons with bipolar disorder. One early study examined the effects of medication plus a six-session CBT protocol focusing on medication adherence (for lithium treatment) (Cochran, 1984). The combined treatment group demonstrated significantly better adherence with lithium and fewer hospitalizations over a six-month follow-up period than the lithium-only group. Another study examined the specific effects of teaching patients to recognize early mood symptoms and then generating strategies for immediate interventions to prevent further symptom acceleration. This intervention was associated with 30 percent fewer manic relapses, greater time well before experiencing manic relapse, and significantly better social functioning over an 18-month follow-up period. However, this specific CBT intervention, which focused on medication adherence, was less effective in reducing depressive relapses (Perry, Tarrier, Morriss, McCarthy, & Limb, 1999).

Several studies have compared cognitive behavioral approaches plus pharmacotherapy to "usual care" plus pharmacotherapy. A 2003 study randomized 103 patients with bipolar disorder to receive either CBT or serve in a control condition (Lam, Watkins, & Hayward, 2003). Both groups received minimal psychiatric care, defined as mood stabilizers at a recommended level and routine psychiatric follow-up. The CBT group received an average of 14 sessions of cognitive therapy during the first six months and two booster sessions in the final six months of the study, with a focus on reducing depression symptoms as well as preventing new mood episodes. Results indicate that those in the CBT group experienced significantly fewer mood episodes and symptoms over the 12-month period. However, 30-month follow-up indicates that the effect for relapse prevention was primarily limited to the first year, and booster sessions or maintenance approaches may be necessary to maintain the benefits of CBT (Lam, Hayward, Watkins, Wright, & Sham, 2005). A smaller study conducted in Australia confirmed the immediate benefits of CBT and the need to explore ways to preserve maintenance of these skills, once learned (Ball et al., 2006).

As discussed in the section on psychoeducational interventions, education may be multifaceted and could include ongoing symptom monitoring for early detection and interventions for emergent mood symptoms, coping with symptoms and consequences of bipolar disorder, and improving psychosocial problem management.

A more recent trial, which enrolled a broader patient population, did not support the benefits of CBT. This study was a multicenter trial for 253 bipolar patients treated at community mental health centers in the United Kingdom (Scott et al., 2006). Patients were randomized to 22 sessions of CBT and pharmacotherapy or usual care and pharmacotherapy. Importantly, in this trial, patients could enter in any clinical state (recovered, subsyndromal, or syndromal). There were no differential effects of CBT and pharmacotherapy on time to recurrence over an 18-month follow-up. Patients with fewer than 12 prior illness episodes had fewer recurrences in CBT than in treatment-as-usual, suggesting that CBT may be more appropriate for patients in the early stages of their disorder or for those with less severe course of illness and comorbidity.

In a different application, CBT was used as maintenance therapy for 79 fully remitted or minimally symptomatic bipolar I and II patients on stable medications (Zaretsky, Rizvi, & Parikh, 2007; Zaretsky, Lance, Miller, Harris, & Parikh, 2008). Seven sessions of psychoeducation plus 13 sessions of CBT were compared to psychoeducation alone. While rates of relapse were similar across the two groups (CBT+psychoeducation compared to psychoeducation alone), those who received add-on CBT experienced 50 percent fewer depressed days and fewer increases in antidepressant medications over the 12-month study follow-up.

While the evidence in support of CBT is somewhat mixed, the studies include diverse subject samples and differences in the content of interventions. The immediate benefit of CBT-based interventions appears clear, and further research to explore patient populations who are most likely to benefit from CBT, as well as ways to maintain and prolong observed benefits, is needed.

IPSRT Strategies

Interpersonal Social Rhythm Therapy (IPSRT) is a short-term and present-focused, individual therapy derived from the interpersonal psychosocial therapy used to treat depression (Klerman, Weissman, Rounsaville, & Chevron, 1984; Weissman, Markowitz, & Klerman, 2000). The philosophy of traditional interpersonal therapy is that, for individuals genetically prone to bipolar disorder, stressful interpersonal events may contribute to the onset of symptoms, **particularly depressive symptoms**. Thus, this approach focuses on the interpersonal context in which symptoms emerge. Patients learn to identify problematic social patterns and relate changes in their moods to these patterns.

Clinicians help patients determine which of the following core problem areas may be contributing to their symptoms:

Although an IPSRT-based theoretical intervention package includes some elements of psychoeducation, it focuses on interpersonal contexts in which symptoms (particularly depression symptoms) emerge, helping patients identify problematic social patterns and relate their moods to these patterns. This focus is what differentiates IPSRT from a strictly psychoeducational approach to treatment.

- ▶ Grief over loss (including "grieving the lost healthy self")
- ▶ Interpersonal conflicts
- ▶ Role transitions
- ▶ Interpersonal skills deficits

Patients then learn ways to resolve current problems and strategies to prevent their reemergence.

Grief over Loss (Including "Grieving the Lost Healthy Self")

The clinician assesses for the presence of *abnormal grief*. In some cases, this form of grief includes grieving over the lost "healthy" self or opportunities missed due to illness. For example, a person who experienced their first debilitating symptoms as a student may grieve never finishing college. Abnormal grief can also include delayed grief responses, in which a person grieves long after the loss. For example, a patient who has recently had a birthday may experience new and profound grief over the death of her own mother, who died at the same age 20 years previously.

abnormal grief—acute grief persisting beyond the typical two to four months that may contribute to depressive symptoms or exacerbate a bipolar depressive episode

Treatment goals associated with grief center on facilitating the mourning process and helping the patient reestablish interests and relationships that can substitute for what has been lost.

Interpersonal Conflicts

The patient and a significant other may have ongoing conflicting expectations about their relationship that may contribute to the development or worsening of symptoms. Treatment goals include identifying the disputes, making choices about a plan of action, and then modifying communication patterns and/or reassessing expectations to resolve the dispute. For example, an unemployed person with bipolar disorder may have accumulated significant debt from previous spending sprees while symptomatic and expect family members to resolve those debts. This results in ongoing conflict and arguments with family members. In this situation, the patient may work with the clinician to improve communication and persuasion skills, so that he can discuss expectations and needs with his family in a reasonable and successful way. Alternatively, the patient may revise expectations and begin to work toward resolving the financial problems through other means.

Role Transitions (Changes in One's Job or Family Situation)

When a person has difficulty coping with life changes that require a role change, the clinician will work with the patient to give up a previous role; express anger, guilt, or loss; acquire new skills; and develop new attachments and support groups. For example, a person may experience a divorce and have mood symptoms as a consequence of dissatisfaction with their changed relationship status. The clinician and patient may work together to recognize the positive aspects of single life and the dissolution of an unhappy marriage, enhance the person's social contacts, and acclimate to this role change.

Interpersonal Skill Deficits

The interpersonal therapy model predicts that interpersonal deficits (e.g., poor conversational skills, dependence) can contribute to mood symptoms. This area of treatment seeks to reduce social isolation and help the patient acquire skills to build intimate and lasting relationships. The clinician may help the patient identify the characteristics of previously successful relationships, such as those built around shared interests (e.g., woodworking, pottery, travel). The clinician may then suggest enrolling in a related class or joining a special interest group to improve the patient's social interactions.

Especially important for bipolar disorder, IPSRT focuses on the role of stressful life events on a patient's social and circadian rhythms. The underlying premise is that symptoms may result from changes in sleep routines, changes in social stimulation, and neurotransmitter dysregulation. Patients learn to monitor the interrelations between their daily routines, sleep, levels of social stimulation, and mood as well as how a change in one domain affects others. For example, a patient may recognize that he tends to experience emergent hypomanic symptoms when he sleeps irregularly, or less than eight hours per night. When generating possible solutions to that pattern, the patient may consider using prescribed medications, a warm bath at bedtime, or other interventions to ensure getting eight hours of sleep each night.

In later phases of treatment, patients work toward regulating their daily routines and sleep/wake cycles and finding optimal balance. They also learn to anticipate and develop plans for coping with events that might be disruptive to established routines. For example, a shift worker may work with the clinician to cope with the supervisor's occasional requests that he work a double shift that could potentially disrupt his sleep-wake routine. He may rehearse an appropriate response to that request, respectfully declining the extra hours.

Effectiveness of IPSRT

A large maintenance trial based at the University of Pittsburgh studied the effectiveness of IPSRT in addition to pharmacotherapy versus intensive clinical management (ICM) plus pharmacotherapy (Frank et al., 2005). ICM group participants attended one-on-one sessions with a clinician, but the content of those meetings was limited to discussion of symptoms, education, medication adherence, and management of side effects. Study authors describe ICM as "low-dose" psychosocial therapy, compared to the more intensive, "high-dose" psychosocial inter-

Those with long histories of inadequate or superficial interpersonal relationships may have deficits that lead to social isolation.

These interventions are individually tailored to the needs of the specific patient, but are designed to protect and preserve essential social rhythms and routines. For example, when attending a family reunion with many people, high levels of social stimulation, and changes in routine and schedule, the person with bipolar disorder may reserve a room in a nearby hotel, to allow time away from the intense social atmosphere for rest and renewal.

In addition, IPSRT may help promote euthymic periods for those with bipolar disorder (Frank et al., 1997).

vention of IPSRT (Frank et al., 2000). Although there were no differences between groups in rates of stabilization during the acute phase, those in IPSRT had longer survival times (without recurrence) during the maintenance phase of the study, regardless of whether they received IPSRT during the maintenance period. Moreover, patients who received IPSRT were more able to regulate their social routines and sleep-wake cycles during the acute phase, and this was associated with fewer recurrences during maintenance treatment. Thus, IPSRT was an effective preventive treatment and, consistent with its hypothesized mechanisms, appeared to operate through the stabilization of social rhythms.

One small open trial ($n = 30$) combined family psychoeducation and individually administered IPSRT with pharmacotherapy (IFIT, Integrated Family and Individual Therapy; Miklowitz et al., 2003). Patient outcomes were compared to those achieved by a comparison group that received two family psychoeducation sessions, pharmacotherapy, and crisis management in a previous trial. Over one year, patients in the IFIT group experienced longer intervals of wellness (42.5 weeks compared to 34.5 weeks) and experienced greater reduction in severity of depressive symptoms than patients in the historical comparison group. The effects were not attributable to differences in medication regimens or adherence.

Which Psychosocial Approaches Are Best for the Treatment of Bipolar Disorder?

Comparisons of Different Therapeutic Approaches

One large study ($n = 293$) compared adjunctive intensive psychotherapy (IPSRT, CBT, or FFT) to collaborative care, a three-session psychoeducation program (Miklowitz et al., 2007) in depressed outpatients with bipolar disorder diagnoses. Patients who received intensive psychotherapy had significantly higher recovery rates after one year (64.4 percent) than those in collaborative care (51.5 percent). While the study was not powered to detect differences in intensive psychotherapy approaches, rates of recovery in each group were 77 percent FFT, 65 percent IPSRT, and 60 percent from CBT.

A recent review compiled findings from 14 randomized trials of various psychotherapy approaches for bipolar disorder (Miklowitz, 2008). The author concluded that treatments focused on early identification of symptoms and treatment adherence have greater effects in reduction or prevention of manic episodes, while treatments that focused on cognitive or inter-personal strategies were more effective against depressive episodes.

Adding psychosocial interventions to pharmacological treatments may optimize bipolar disorder treatment by:

- ▶ Substantially improving medication adherence
- ▶ Optimizing clinical and functional outcomes
- ▶ Increasing periods of wellness between mood episodes
- ▶ Improving overall quality of life and satisfaction with treatment

As with all interventions, the choice to add psychosocial interventions should be carefully weighed through conversation between care provider and patient, considering both the potential positive effects as well as possible risks. Two potential risks of increased awareness and knowledge about the disorder are the following (Gonzalez-Pinto et al., 2004):

1. Greater awareness of depressive symptoms and early symptom detection has been linked with increased antidepressant use, with no associated reduction in depressive episodes (Perry et al., 1999). Therefore, education should also include instruction in alternate coping strategies for depressive symptoms.

2. Having greater knowledge of the disorder has been associated with increased anxiety during the early phases of treatment (Van Gent & Zwart, 1991). This can be alleviated by providing appropriate reassurance and pharmacological support as necessary.

It has been suggested that future research focus on identifying neurobiological markers of response to psychotherapy and tailoring specific interventions to subtypes of illness course and characteristics (Vieta et al., 2009; Miklowitz, 2008). Further research is needed on the mechanisms of psychosocial interventions, including what aspects are most important to obtain positive results, to further understand how to best combine treatments for individuals with bipolar disorder.

Key Concepts for Chapter 4

1. Research demonstrates that psychosocial interventions are helpful adjuncts to traditional pharmacological treatment of bipolar disorder. Psychosocial interventions can reduce acute symptoms, prevent new episodes, increase adherence with medication, and decrease rates of hospitalization.

2. Psychosocial interventions can help teach patients strategies to improve coping with stressful life events, increase social support networks, regularize sleep-wake cycles, and identify and control psychological mechanisms that may exacerbate bipolar illness.

3. Most psychosocial interventions are diverse and employ a variety of techniques and interventions based on the unique needs of an individual.

4. Most psychosocial treatment packages include some form of psychoeducation. A number of structured psychoeducational interventions have demonstrated effectiveness in teaching patients and family members about bipolar disorder, treatment options, the importance of adherence, and prevention of relapse. These interventions can help prolong periods of wellness for individuals with bipolar disorder.

5. Therapies with research evidence to support their effectiveness for patients with bipolar disorder include family-focused therapy (FFT), cognitive-behavioral therapies (CBT), and interpersonal social rhythm therapy (IPSRT).

Appendix A
DSM-IV–TR Diagnostic Criteria

Criteria for Major Depressive Episode

A. Five (or more) of the following symptoms have been present during the same 2-week period and represent a change from previous functioning; at least one of the symptoms is either (1) depressed mood or (2) loss of interest or pleasure.

Note: Do not include symptoms that are clearly due to a general medical condition, or mood-incongruent delusions or hallucinations.

(1) Depressed mood most of the day, nearly every day, as indicated by either subjective report (e.g., feels sad or empty) or observation made by others (e.g., appears tearful). **Note:** In children and adolescents, can be irritable mood.

(2) Markedly diminished interest or pleasure in all, or almost all, activities most of the day, nearly every day (as indicated by either subjective account or observation made by others)

(3) Significant weight loss when not dieting or weight gain (e.g., a change of more than 5 percent of body weight in a month), or decrease or increase in appetite nearly every day. **Note:** In children, consider failure to make expected weight gains.

(4) Insomnia or hypersomnia nearly every day

(5) Psychomotor agitation or retardation nearly every day (observable by others, not merely subjective feelings of restlessness or being slowed down)

(6) Fatigue or loss of energy nearly every day

(7) Feelings of worthlessness or excessive or inappropriate guilt (which may be delusional) nearly every day (not merely self-reproach or guilt about being sick)

(8) Diminished ability to think or concentrate, or indecisiveness, nearly every day (either by subjective account or as observed by others)

(9) Recurrent thoughts of death (not just fear of dying), recurrent suicidal ideation without a specific plan, or a suicide attempt or a specific plan for committing suicide

This appendix presents diagnostic criteria relevant for bipolar disorder assessment, reprinted with permission from the American Psychological Association, as follows:

▶ *Criteria for Major Depressive Episode*

▶ *Criteria for Manic Episode*

▶ *Criteria for Mixed Episode*

▶ *Criteria for Hypomanic Episode*

▶ *Diagnostic Criteria for 296.0x Bipolar I Disorder, Single Manic Episode*

▶ *Diagnostic Criteria for 296.40 Bipolar I Disorder, Most Recent Episode Hypomanic*

▶ *Diagnostic Criteria for 296.4x Bipolar I Disorder, Most Recent Episode Manic*

▶ *Diagnostic Criteria for 296.5x Bipolar I Disorder, Most Recent Episode Depressed*

▶ *Diagnostic Criteria for 296.6x Bipolar I Disorder, Most Recent Episode Mixed*

▶ *Diagnostic Criteria for 296.7 Bipolar I Disorder, Most Recent Episode Unspecified*

▶ *Diagnostic Criteria for 296.89 Bipolar II Disorder*

▶ *Diagnostic Criteria for 301.13 Cyclothymic Disorder*

B. The symptoms do not meet criteria for a Mixed Episode.

C. The symptoms cause clinically significant distress or impairment in social, occupational, or other important areas of functioning.

D. The symptoms are not due to the direct physiological effects of a substance (e.g., a drug of abuse, a medication) or a general medical condition (e.g., hypothyroidism).

E. The symptoms are not better accounted for by Bereavement, i.e., after the loss of a loved one, the symptoms persist for longer than 2 months or are characterized by marked functional impairment, morbid preoccupation with worthlessness, suicidal ideation, psychotic symptoms, or psychomotor retardation.

Criteria for Manic Episode

A. A distinct period of abnormally and persistently elevated, expansive, or irritable mood, lasting at least 1 week (or any duration if hospitalization is necessary).

B. During the period of mood disturbance, three (or more) of the following symptoms have persisted (four if the mood is only irritable) and have been present to a significant degree:

    (1)   Inflated self-esteem or grandiosity

    (2)   Decreased need for sleep (e.g., feels rested after only 3 hours of sleep)

    (3)   More talkative than usual or pressure to keep talking

    (4)   Flight of ideas or subjective experience that thoughts are racing

    (5)   Distractibility (i.e., attention too easily drawn to unimportant or irrelevant external stimuli)

    (6)   Increase in goal-directed activity (either socially, at work or school, or sexually) or psychomotor agitation

    (7)   Excessive involvement in pleasurable activities that have a high potential for painful consequences (e.g., engaging in unrestrained buying sprees, sexual indiscretions, or foolish investments)

C. The symptoms do not meet criteria for a Mixed Episode.

D. The mood disturbance is sufficiently severe to cause marked impairment in occupational functioning or in usual social activities or relationships with others, or to necessitate hospitalization to prevent harm to self or others, or there are psychotic features.

E. The symptoms are not due to the direct physiological effects of a substance (e.g., a drug of abuse, a medication, or other treatment) or a general medical condition (e.g., hyperthyroidism). **Note:** Manic-like episodes that are clearly caused by somatic antidepressant treatment (e.g., medication, electroconvulsive therapy, light therapy) should not count toward a diagnosis of Bipolar I Disorder.

Criteria for Mixed Episode

A. The criteria are met both for a Manic Episode and for a Major Depressive Episode (except for duration) nearly every day during at least a 1-week period.

B. The mood disturbance is sufficiently severe to cause marked impairment inoccupational functioning or in usual social activities or relationships with others, or to necessitate hospitalization to prevent harm to self or others, or there are psychotic features.

C. The symptoms are not due to the direct physiological effects of a substance (e.g., a drug of abuse, a medication, or other treatment) or a general medical condition (e.g., hyperthyroidism).

Note: Mixed-like episodes that are clearly caused by somatic antidepressant treatment (e.g., medication, electroconvulsive therapy, light therapy) should not count toward a diagnosis of Bipolar I Disorder.

Criteria for Hypomanic Episode

A. A distinct period of persistently elevated, expansive, or irritable mood, lasting throughout at least 4 days, that is clearly different from the usual nondepressed mood.

B. During the period of mood disturbance, three (or more) of the following symptoms have persisted (four if the mood is only irritable) and have been present to a significant degree:

(1) Inflated self-esteem or grandiosity

(2) Decreased need for sleep (e.g., feels rested after only 3 hours of sleep)

(3) More talkative than usual or pressure to keep talking

(4) Flight of ideas or subjective experience that thoughts are racing

(5) Distractibility (i.e., attention too easily drawn to unimportant or irrelevant external stimuli)

(6) Increase in goal-directed activity (either socially, at work or school, or sexually) or psychomotor agitation

(7) Excessive involvement in pleasurable activities that have a high potential for painful consequences (e.g., the person engages in unrestrained buying sprees, sexual indiscretions, or foolish business investments)

C. The episode is associated with an unequivocal change in functioning that is uncharacteristic of the person when not symptomatic.

D. The disturbance in mood and the change in functioning are observable by others.

E. The episode is not severe enough to cause marked impairment in social or occupational functioning, or to necessitate hospitalization, and there are no psychotic features.

F. The symptoms are not due to the direct physiological effects of a substance (e.g., a drug of abuse, a medication, or other treatment) or a general medical condition (e.g., hyperthyroidism). **Note:** Hypomanic-like episodes that are clearly caused by somatic antidepressant treatment (e.g., medication, electroconvulsive therapy, light therapy) should not count toward a diagnosis of Bipolar II Disorder.

Diagnostic Criteria for 296.0x Bipolar I Disorder, Single Manic Episode

A. Presence of only one Manic Episode and no past Major Depressive Episodes. **Note:** Recurrence is defined as either a change in polarity from depression or an interval of at least 2 months without manic symptoms.

B. The Manic Episode is not better accounted for by Schizoaffective Disorder and is not superimposed on Schizophrenia, Schizophreniform Disorder, Delusional Disorder, or Psychotic Disorder Not Otherwise Specified.

Specify if:

Mixed: if symptoms meet criteria for a Mixed Episode

If the full criteria are currently met for a Manic, Mixed, or Major Depressive Episode, specify its current clinical status and/or features:

Mild, Moderate, Severe Without Psychotic Features/Severe With Psychotic Features

With Catatonic Features

With Postpartum Onset

If the full criteria are not currently met for a Manic, Mixed, or Major Depressive Episode, specify the current clinical status of the Bipolar I Disorder or features of the most recent episode:

In Partial Remission, In Full Remission

With Catatonic Features

With Postpartum Onset

Diagnostic Criteria for 296.40 Bipolar I Disorder, Most Recent Episode Hypomanic

A. Currently (or most recently) in a Hypomanic Episode

B. There has previously been at least one Manic Episode or Mixed Episode.

C. The mood symptoms cause clinically significant distress or impairment in social, occupational, or other important areas of functioning.

D. The mood episodes in Criteria A and B are not better accounted for by Schizoaffective Disorder and are not superimposed on Schizophrenia, Schizophreniform Disorder, Delusional Disorder, or Psychotic Disorder Not Otherwise Specified.

Specify:

Longitudinal Course Specifiers (With and Without Interepisode Recovery)

With Seasonal Pattern (applies only to the pattern of Major Depressive Episodes)

With Rapid Cycling

Diagnostic Criteria for 296.4x Bipolar I Disorder, Most Recent Episode Manic

A. Currently (or most recently) in a Manic Episode

B. There has previously been at least one Major Depressive Episode, Manic Episode, or Mixed Episode.

C. The mood episodes in Criteria A and B are not better accounted for by Schizoaffective Disorder and are not superimposed on Schizophrenia, Schizophreniform Disorder, Delusional Disorder, or Psychotic Disorder Not Otherwise Specified.

If the full criteria are currently met for a Manic Episode, specify its current clinical status and/or features:

Mild, Moderate, Severe Without Psychotic Features/Severe With Psychotic Features

With Catatonic Features

With Postpartum Onset

If the full criteria are not currently met for a Manic Episode, specify its current clinical status of the Bipolar I Disorder and/ or features of the most recent Manic Episode:

In Partial Remission, In Full Remission

With Catatonic Features

With Postpartum Onset

Specify:

Longitudinal Course Specifiers (With and Without Interepisode Recovery)

With Seasonal Pattern (applies only to the pattern of Major Depressive Episodes)

With Rapid Cycling

Diagnostic Criteria for 296.6x Bipolar I Disorder, Most Recent Episode Mixed

A. Currently (or most recently) in a Mixed Episode

B. There has previously been at least one Major Depressive Episode, Manic Episode, or Mixed Episode.

C. The mood episodes in Criteria A and B are not better accounted for by Schizoaffective Disorder and are not superimposed on Schizophrenia, Schizophreniform Disorder, Delusional Disorder, or Psychotic Disorder Not Otherwise Specified.

If the full criteria are currently met for a Mixed Episode, specify its current clinical status and/or features:

Mild, Moderate, Severe Without Psychotic Features/Severe With Psychotic Features

With Catatonic Features

With Postpartum Onset

If the full criteria are not currently met for a Mixed Episode, specify its current clinical status of the Bipolar I Disorder and/or features of the most recent Mixed Episode:

In Partial Remission, In Full Remission

With Catatonic Features

With Postpartum Onset

Specify:

Longitudinal Course Specifiers (With and Without Interepisode Recovery

With Seasonal Pattern (applies only to the pattern of Major Depressive Episodes)

With Rapid Cycling

Diagnostic Criteria for 296.5x Bipolar I Disorder, Most Recent Episode Depressed

A. Currently (or most recently) in a Major Depressive Episode

B. There has previously been at least one Manic Episode, Mixed Episode

C. The mood episodes in Criteria A and B are not better accounted for by Schizoaffective Disorder and are not superimposed on Schizophrenia, Schizophreniform Disorder, Delusional Disorder, or Psychotic Disorder Not Otherwise Specified.

If the full criteria are currently met for a Major Depressive Episode, specify its current clinical status and/or features:

    Mild, Moderate, Severe Without Psychotic Features/Severe With Psychotic Features

    Chronic

    With Catatonic Features

    With Melancholic Features

    With Atypical Features

    With Postpartum Onset

If the full criteria are currently met for a Major Depressive Episode, specify the current clinical status of the Bipolar I Disorder and/or features of the most recent Major Depressive Episode:

    In Partial Remission, In Full Remission

    Chronic

    With Catatonic Features

    With Melancholic Features

    With Atypical Features

    With Postpartum Onset

Specify:

    Longitudinal Course Specifiers (With and Without Interepisode Recovery)

    With Seasonal Pattern (applies only to the pattern of Major Depressive Episodes)

    With Rapid Cycling

Diagnostic Criteria for 296.7 Bipolar I Disorder, Most Recent Episode Unspecified

A. Criteria, except for duration, are currently (or most recently) met for a Manic, a Hypomanic, a Mixed, or a Major Depressive Episode

B. There has previously been at least one Manic Episode or Mixed Episode.

C. The mood symptoms cause clinically significant distress or impairment in social, occupational, or other important areas of functioning.

D. The mood symptoms in Criteria A and B are not better accounted for by Schizoaffective Disorder and are not superimposed on Schizophrenia, Schizophreniform Disorder, Delusional Disorder, or Psychotic Disorder Not Otherwise Specified.

E. The mood symptoms in Criteria A and B are not due to the direct physiological effects of a substance (e.g., a drug of abuse, a medication, or other treatment) or a general medical condition (e.g., hyperthyroidism).

Specify:

Longitudinal Course Specifiers (With and Without Interepisode Recovery)

With Seasonal Pattern (applies only to the pattern of Major Depressive Episodes)

With Rapid Cycling

Diagnostic Criteria for 296.89 Bipolar II Disorder

A. Presence (or history) of one or more Major Depressive Episodes

B. Presence (or history) of at least one Hypomanic Episode

C. There has never been a Manic Episode or a Mixed Episode

D. The mood symptoms in Criteria A and B are not better accounted for by Schizoaffective Disorder and are not superimposed on Schizophrenia, Schizophreniform Disorder, Delusional Disorder, or Psychotic Disorder Not Otherwise Specified.

E. The symptoms cause clinically significant distress or impairment in social, occupational, or other important areas of functioning.

Specify current or most recent episode:

Hypomanic: if currently (or most recently) in a Hypomanic Episode

Depressed: if currently (or most recently) in a Major Depressive Episode

If the full criteria are currently met for a Major Depressive Episode, specify its current clinical status and/or features:

Mild, Moderate, Severe Without Psychotic Features/Severe With Psychotic Features

Note: Fifth-digit codes specified cannot be used here because the code for Bipolar II Disorder already uses the fifth digit.

Chronic

With Catatonic Features

With Melancholic Features

With Atypical Features

With Postpartum Onset

If the full criteria are currently met for a Hypomanic or Major Depressive Episode, specify its clinical status of the Bipolar II Disorder and/or features of the most recent Major Depressive Episode (only if it is the most recent type of mood episode):

In Partial Remission, In Full Remission

Note: Fifth-digit codes specified cannot be used here because the code for Bipolar II Disorder already uses the fifth digit.

Chronic

With Catatonic Features

With Melancholic Features

With Atypical Features

With Postpartum Onset

Specify:

Longitudinal Course Specifiers (With and Without Interepisode Recovery)

With Seasonal Pattern (applies only to the pattern of Major Depressive Episodes)

With Rapid Cycling

Diagnostic Criteria for 301.13 Cyclothymic Disorder

A. For at least 2 years, the presence of numerous periods with hypomanic symptoms and numerous periods with depressive symptoms that do not meet criteria for a Major Depressive Episode.

Note: In children and adolescents, the duration must be at least 1 year.

B. During the above 2-year period (1 year in children and adolescents), the person has not been without the symptoms in Criterion A for more than 2 months at a time.

C. No Major Depressive Episode, Manic Episode, or Mixed Episode has been present during the first 2 years of the disturbance.

Note: After the initial 2 years (1 year in children and adolescents) of Cyclothymic Disorder, there may be superimposed Manic or Mixed Episodes (in which case both Bipolar I Disorder and Cyclothymic Disorder may be diagnosed) or Major Depressive Episodes (in which case both Bipolar II Disorder and Cyclothymic Disorder may be diagnosed).

D. The symptoms in Criteria A are not better accounted for by Schizoaffective Disorder and are not superimposed on Schizophrenia, Schizophreniform Disorder, Delusional Disorder, or Psychotic Disorder Not Otherwise Specified.

E. The symptoms are not due to the direct physiological effects of a substance (e.g., a drug of abuse, a medication) or a general medical condition (e.g., hyperthyroidism).

F. The symptoms cause clinically significant distress or impairment in social, occupational, or other important areas of functioning.

Appendix B
Tools for Diagnosis and Assessment of Bipolar Disorder

Diagnosis of Bipolar Disorders

Structured Clinical Interviews

 LINICAL interviewing tools for diagnosing bipolar disorder include:

- ► The Schedule for Affective Disorders and Schizophrenia (SADS)
- ► Diagnostic Interview Schedule (DIS)
- ► The Structured Clinical Interview for the *DSM-IV* (SCID)

SADS

Developed to differentiate between affective disorders and schizophrenia, the SADS must be administered by trained professionals. It is designed to evaluate current and lifetime affective disorders and yields diagnoses consistent with research criteria for bipolar disorder, depression, and other diagnostic categories.

The instrument is a semi-structured interview divided into two parts.

- ► Part I obtains a detailed description of the clinical features of the current episode and during the week prior to the interview.
- ► Part II obtains historical information needed to confirm a lifetime diagnosis. It also provides estimates of severity.

Questions are progressive and have built-in criteria for whether or not to rule out the symptoms for current diagnostic purposes.

DIS

The DIS is a highly structured, diagnostic interview designed to be administered by experienced lay interviewers without clinical training (Robins et al., 1996). The DIS has been used in psychiatric survey research for decades to assess the prevalence of psychiatric disorders in the general population. Modules cover mood, anxiety, schizophrenia, eating, *somatization,* psychoactive substance abuse, and antisocial personality disorders. The DIS provides both current and lifetime diagnostic information. Its content directly corresponds to DSM-IV-TR diagnostic criteria.

Overall, the regular SADS has demonstrated excellent reliability, particularly for interrater and test-retest reliabilities related to current episodes of psychiatric disturbance.

somatization—multiple physical complaints involving any body system

The computerized version can be self-administered with the availability of an assistant to answer questions if needed. Research shows that professionals and paraprofessionals using the DIS reach compatible diagnoses (Helzer, Spitznagel, & McEvoy, 1987).

Data on the reliability of diagnosis using the DIS versus clinical judgment is variable. This is expected, based upon the problems of relying on psychiatrist ratings as the "gold standard" of diagnosis. It has been suggested that these data be considered a form of interrater reliability, versus concurrent validity.

SCID

The SCID is a structured, broad-spectrum instrument that adheres closely to the *DSM-IV* decision trees for psychiatric diagnosis (First et al., 1997). There are multiple versions, including a briefer clinical version, a research version, and a module to assess for the presence of personality disorders. The SCID is designed for use by trained interviewers to ensure a structured and consistent format for investigating psychiatric symptoms.

The SCID and its variations include some open-ended questions and a skip pattern (i.e., negative responses to certain questions cause the interviewer to skip ahead in the instrument), which results in a shorter administration time for those with fewer symptoms. Trained professional interviewers administer the SCID, as clinical judgment is required throughout the interview.

Research on the reliability of the SCID has found variable test-retest and interrater reliabilities, varying by diagnostic categories. Validity studies of the SCID have assumed that *DSM*-based diagnostic categories are the benchmark for making comparisons of diagnostic accuracy. Thus, "procedural validity" is assumed, as the SCID closely mirrors the criteria specified in *DSM* versions (Rogers, 1995).

Self-Report Screening Instrument for Bipolar Disorders

Mood Disorders Questionnaire (MDQ)

The MDQ is a brief, self-administered diagnostic screening instrument (Hirschfeld et al., 2000). While it screens for the presence or absence of symptoms consistent with a bipolar diagnosis, it provides no information about the severity and duration of those symptoms. As with all self-report instruments, it is also dependent on the person's awareness of symptoms and experiences. It includes 13 "yes/no" items derived from both

DSM-IV criteria and clinical experience. A positive screen requires that:

▶ Seven or more items must be endorsed.

▶ Several of the items must co-occur.

▶ The symptoms cause at least moderate psychosocial impairment.

The instrument demonstrated good *sensitivity* (0.73) and very good *specificity* (0.90) in outpatients treated at five outpatient psychiatric clinics. It has also been validated in an adolescent outpatient psychiatry population (Wagner et al., 2006). In contrast, when tested in a national epidemiological sample, the instrument correctly identified only 28.1 percent (weighted sensitivity) of those with SCID diagnoses on the bipolar spectrum (Hirschfeld et al., 2003). In the same sample, the MDQ identified 97.2 percent of individuals without bipolar disorder as "not bipolar" (weighted specificity). This scale may be a useful adjunct to other assessments because it is brief, and patients can complete it independently in the waiting room. However, diagnostic decisions cannot be made based on the MDQ alone.

sensitivity—the degree to which the instrument correctly identifies patients that **do have** the disorder

specificity—the degree to which the instrument correctly identifies patients that **do not have** the disorder

Assessment of Symptoms

Clinician-Administered Observational Rating Scales

A number of assessment tools involve a combination of structured to semi-structured interview and behavioral observations, designed for administration by a trained interviewer. Training is essential to avoid the following possible distortions in clinician-rated assessment:

▶ Interviewer bias, in which an interviewer systematically rates in a certain direction (e.g., rating the patient as more severely ill to justify continued treatment)

▶ Differences in administration of the scale, which can impact the applicability of results

▶ Variations in the interview environment (interviewer and patient mood, distractions, behavior, etc.) which might alter results

Clinician-administered instruments used to assess the presence and severity of manic symptoms include the Young Mania Rating Scale (YMRS) and the Clinician Administered Rating Scale for Mania (CARS-M).

YMRS

This 11-item measure was designed to measure the severity of manic symptoms and to detect the effects of treatment on mania

interrater reliability—degree to which different raters agree on a diagnosis based on the use of the instrument

interitem reliability—degree to which scores on individual items agree with each other; an estimate of the extent to which the instrument is measuring a single construct.

(Young et al., 1978). It includes both mild and severe versions of manic symptoms. Items are ranked on a scale of 0–4 or 0–8. Professionals can administer the YMRS after minimal training.

The YMRS has demonstrated good *interrater* and *interitem reliability,* and it has a strong association to other measures of manic symptoms. It is typically utilized as the "gold standard" measurement of manic symptoms in research settings.

CARS-M

The CARS-M was designed to evaluate the severity of manic and psychotic symptoms and to detect changes in such symptoms over the course of treatment (Altman et al., 1994). It includes two subscales that are individually scored, measuring mania and psychosis, respectively. Items assessing mania were derived from the SADS, described above. The scale includes 15 items that are rated from 0 to 6 on a Likert scale, except for one item, insight, which is rated 0–4. Each item has anchors, and the scale also includes prompts to aid clinicians in probing certain symptom domains. Clinicians are also permitted to use collateral information, such as family and medical histories, when making ratings.

Reliability for the CARS-M is substantial (Altman et al., 1994). Additionally, the CARS-M correlates strongly (0.94) with the YMRS. Research evidence suggests that the manic subscale can differentiate manic patients from those with other severe psychiatric disturbances (Altman et al., 1994).

Clinician-rated scales used to assess depressive symptoms include the Hamilton Rating Scale for Depression (HAM-D), Montgomery-Äsberg Depression Rating Scale (MADRS), and the Inventory of Depressive Symptomatology–Clinician Rated (IDS-C) or its brief version, the Quick Inventory of Depressive Symptomatology–Clinician Rated (QIDS-C).

HAM-D

The HAM-D is also available in a computerized version and a paper-and-pencil, self-report version.

The HAM-D was initially created to assess depression severity in those already diagnosed (Hamilton, 1960, 1967; Williams, 1988). It has become a common outcome measure for evaluating the effects of different treatment interventions. The HAM-D is a 21-item scale completed during a 30-minute interview (only the first 17 items are scored, thus the scale is often referred to as the "HAM-17"). It includes a checklist of symptoms ranked on a scale of 0–4 or 0–2 and was designed to be administered by physicians, psychologists, and social workers who have experience with psychiatric populations. However, the HAM-D can be administered by nonclinicians after some training.

The internal consistency is higher with use of the structured interview form (Potts, Daniels, Burnam, & Wells, 1990). Reports of interrater reliability have been consistent and high, ranging from 0.65 to 0.9 for the total score. Results from the HAM-D are highly correlated with results from other observer-rated instruments, such as the MADRS and IDS, and range from 0.80 to 0.90.

MADRS

The MADRS is a clinician-rated measure which provides data on overall depression severity and specific depressive symptoms (Davidson et al., 1986; Kearns et al., 1982; Montgomery & Äsberg, 1979). It has been demonstrated to be sensitive to change in depression symptoms over time. The MADRS includes 10 items, which are rated on a scale of 0–6. Observations as well as verbal information can be incorporated into the ratings.

The reliability of the MADRS is acceptable and comparable to other observer-rated depression scales, with joint reliability for the total scale ranging from 0.76 to 0.95. The following mean scores from the MADRS correspond to global severity measures from the DSM: very severe = 44; severe = 31; moderate = 25; mild = 15; and recovered = 7 (Cassano et al., 2002).

IDS-C

This measure was designed to capture the full range of depressive symptoms and is derived from diagnostic criteria for Major Depressive Disorder found in the *DSM-IV* (Rush et al., 1986; 1996). It includes self-report and clinician-rated forms. It is unique in its efforts to be more comprehensive, including coverage of atypical, melancholic, somatic and cognitive features of depression. The clinician-rated version includes 30 items, which are scored on a four-point anchored scale. It includes a semi-structured interview to assist a trained clinician interviewer.

The IDS-C possesses excellent reliability, achieving an internal consistency of 0.94 in a large sample. It is highly correlated with other depression rating scales.

The QIDS-C (Rush et al., 2003) is a 16-item short version of the IDS-C and includes only nine diagnostic symptom domains used to characterize a major depressive episode, without items to assess atypical, melancholic or other associated symptoms. All 16 items on the QIDS are included within the IDS.

Self-Ratings of Symptoms

Self-ratings are completed independently by the patient and help detect the presence or absence of symptoms. The accuracy of self-rating scales is dependent on the level of insight and recognition of symptoms by the patient. The Life Chart and the ISS are self-report instruments that were developed to capture the entire spectrum of symptoms present in bipolar disorder (Bauer et al., 1991; Denicoff et al., 2000; Leverich & Post, 1998; Post et al., 1988).

Appendix C includes more information and a copy of the Life Chart instructions and sample log.

The Life Chart Method

This tool asks the patient to log daily specific information on mood, sleep, medications, and life events. Copies of a sample log tool are in the public domain and available through the Depression Bipolar Support Alliance (DBSA), www.dbsalliance .org. With clinician assistance, it can also be used to retrospectively retrace the course of illness. This tool can be very helpful for the clinician and the patient to track response to interventions and life events.

ISS

This tool is a 17-item self-report scale that includes assessment of both manic and depressive symptoms. Items are presented as a visual analog scale; respondents mark their response along the scale from 0 to 100. It can be useful in assessing mixed states as well as classic mania and depression. Factor analysis of the ISS reveals four subscales, called Activation, Perceived Conflict, Well-Being, and Depression. The ISS can be completed in approximately 15–20 minutes.

Other Self-Report Scales

Other scales used for assessing symptoms in bipolar disorder include:

▶ **The Altman Mania Rating Scale (AMRS)**—The AMRS (Altman et al., 1997) is a five-item patient self-rating mania scale designed to assess the presence and/or severity of manic symptoms. The AMRS is designed to be a screening instrument, and a diagnosis cannot be reliably made based upon results from this tool. All items are scored from 0 (absent) to 4 (present to a severe degree), based on increasing severity. A cutoff score of 6 or higher on the AMRS indicates a high probability of a manic or hypomanic condition (based on a sensitivity rating of 85.5 percent and a specificity rating of 87.3 percent). A score of 5 or lower is less likely to be associated with significant symptoms of mania. A score of 6 or higher may indicate a need for treatment and/or further diagnostic workup (to confirm a diagnosis of mania or hypomania).

▶ **The IDS-SR**—The IDS-SR (Rush et al., 1986, 1996) is a self-report companion scale to the IDS-C described above. It includes 30 multiple-choice items, with most scored from 0 (least severe) to 3 (most severe). Completion of the IDS-SR requires approximately 15–20 minutes and adequate reading ability. The IDS-SR is highly correlated with other self-report measures of depression (0.93 with the Beck Depression Inventory) and with its companion, clinician-rated version (0.91 with the IDS-C). There is also a shorter 16-item version, the QIDS-SR, which has been validated in patients with bipolar disorder.

▶ **The Beck Depression Inventory (BDI-2)**—The BDI-2 (Beck et al., 1986, 1988) assesses depressive symptoms based on the *DSM-IV* criteria. The patient is asked to respond to 21 items covering specific thoughts and feelings in the areas of cognitive, affective, somatic, and vegetative symptoms of depression experienced within the past week. It is useful for those 13 years and older and can be administered individually or in groups, in a written or oral format. It takes approximately 5–10 minutes to complete and can be scored manually or by computer, with a computer-based interpretation of the scores available. The BDI-2 is intended to be a screening tool for depression, with particular attention to items on hopelessness and suicidal ideation as the best indicators of potential suicidality (Carlson, 1998; Murphy, Impara, & Plake, 1999).

Conducting a General Assessment of Psychiatric Symptoms

A trained clinician might also choose to use a general measure of psychiatric symptoms and/or personality function to assist in the diagnostic process. Although they do not directly assess bipolar symptoms, these measures can be helpful in differentiating symptoms from those associated with other disorders.

BPRS-24

The BPRS-24 is a general measure of psychiatric symptomatology, encompassing a range of symptoms and intended to assess symptom changes in psychiatric patients. This 24-item scale relies on a clinician-administered format, utilizing information gained through behavioral observation and collateral sources (Overall & Gorham, 1988; Ventura et al., 1995).

The initial version (BPRS-18 item) was updated to include three additional items specifically designed to capture manic-phase symptoms for patients with bipolar disorder as well as increased coverage of psychiatric symptoms (Bigelow & Murphy, 1978).

General assessment measures include:

▶ *The Brief Psychiatric Rating Scale (BPRS)*

▶ *The Minnesota Multiphasic Personality Inventory—2nd Edition (MMPI-2)*

▶ *The Millon Clinical Multiaxial Inventory (MCMI-III)*

Items are rated on a 1- to 7-point scale of increasing severity, and the scale is available in a format that incorporates rating anchors and interview probes to enhance interrater reliability and accuracy (Essock, Hargreaves, Covell, & Goethe, 1996).

Good joint reliability is achievable with the BPRS, but it requires thorough training of interviewers. The BPRS has been demonstrated to provide a sensitive, though nonspecific, measure of psychiatric status change. It is correlated with other measures of general psychopathology, and specific items correlate with scales intended to measure the same symptom domain.

MMPI-2

T-scores—standardized scores based on 0 to 100, with a mean of 50

The MMPI-2 is widely used both to assess personality characteristics that may influence response to treatment, and as a general tool to assist with diagnosis and clinical assessment (Butcher et al., 1989). It consists of 567 "true/false" questions, administered in a choice of formats, including an online administration. Results yield *T-scores* for a number of validity, basic, and clinical scales. While the MMPI-2 is a valuable part of the assessment process, particularly with a cooperative patient, understanding the results requires interpretation by a trained professional. Definitive diagnosis cannot be made solely from results on an MMPI-2, but this instrument can be helpful as part of a general diagnostic evaluation, which includes a clinical interview, observation, and other assessment approaches.

Both the MMPI-2 and the MCMI-III are paper-and-pencil, self-administered instruments.

MCMI-III

The MCMI-III was developed to assess clinical personality styles and major clinical syndromes in accordance with Millon's theories of personality and psychopathology as well as *DSM-IV* categories (Millon et al., 1997). It consists of 175 "true/false" items, scored across 24 scales.

While the MCMI-III can be useful as one part of a comprehensive diagnostic evaluation, it is not recommended to rely on solely for diagnostic determinations. The scale is better at identifying personality and psychopathology according to Millon's theoretical model, and less consistent in agreement with DSM-IV diagnostic categories.

Concerns about this instrument include the overlap between scales and the use of base rates in defining cutoff scores for scale interpretation. Individual items can count toward more than one scale, resulting in artificially high correlations between subscales. Additionally, the use of base rates may be inappropriate when the person taking the test is significantly different from those included in the standardization sample.

Appendix C
Life Chart Sample

The Life Chart provides a structure to help patients monitor their moods on a daily basis. The daily and monthly log can also be helpful for the patient and clinician to review response to changes in treatment. The patient completes the log at the end of each day (prior to taking evening medication), recording information about:

- ► Medications taken
- ► Number of hours of sleep from the previous night
- ► Overall mood for the day according to a scale given (if experiencing sudden, distinct, or significant mood changes within the day, patients enter the highest and lowest mood values reached)
- ► The number of mood changes over the course of the day
- ► The severity of mood episodes rated according to level of functional impairment
- ► Whether or not the patient is having a menstrual period (if applicable)
- ► Significant events each day in terms of life events, side effects, and coexisting symptoms

A sample Life Chart log follows on pages 96–97.

MONTH _____   YEAR _____

TOTAL NUMBER OF PILLS TAKEN PER DAY

Days: 1 2 3 4 5 6 7 8 9 10 11 12 13 14 15 16 17 18 19 20 21 22 23 24 25 26 27 28 29 30 31

MEDICATION/SUPPLEMENT NAME — DAILY DOSE — # OF PILLS PER DAY

USED ALCOHOL/DRUGS (✔) IF YES

HOURS OF NIGHTTIME SLEEP

M
A
N
I
A
- SEVERE — Essentially incapacitated or **HOSPITALIZED**
- HIGH MODERATE — GREAT difficulty with goal-oriented activity
- LOW MODERATE — SOME difficulty with goal-oriented activity
- MILD — More energized & productive, usual routine not affected much

STABLE

D
E
P
R
E
S
S
I
O
N
- MILD — Usual routine not affected much
- LOW MODERATE — Functioning with SOME effort
- HIGH MODERATE — Functioning with GREAT effort
- SEVERE — Essentially incapacitated or **HOSPITALIZED**

MIXED STATE (✔) IF YES

MOOD (0 – 10)   -10 •••••••••0•••••••••+10   Most depressed ever   Balanced   Most manic ever

NUMBER OF MOOD CHANGES

ANXIETY SYMPTOMS (✔) IF YES

OTHER SYMPTOMS

INTERFERENCE WITH LIFE (0=LEAST; 10=MOST)

LIFE EVENTS

IMPACT (-10=MOST NEGATIVE; 10=MOST POSITIVE)

1 2 3 4 5 6 7 8 9 10 11 12 13 14 15 16 17 18 19 20 21 22 23 24 25 26 27 28 29 30 31

Glossary

A

abnormal grief—acute grief persisting beyond the typical two to four months that may contribute to depressive symptoms or exacerbate a bipolar depressive episode

absolute starting dose—amount of medication given when the patient first takes it

active listening—a way of listening that focuses entirely on what the other person is saying and confirms understanding of both the message content and the emotions and feelings underlying the message to ensure accurate understanding

affect—the external expression of emotion

algorithms—an organized set of specific recommendations that are evidence-based, often informed by expert consensus opinion when there are inadequate studies to inform treatment decisions

amygdala—one of the basal ganglia that is part of the limbic system and believed to be involved in impulsivity and other functions

assertive communication techniques—these techniques help patients honestly express opinions, feelings, attitudes, and rights (without undue anxiety) in a way that doesn't infringe on the rights of others

attributional style—one's tendencies in making causal explanations about a variety of intra- and interpersonal events in their lives

atypical features—mood reactivity and at least two of the following: increased appetite or weight gain, excessive sleep, the sensation that your limbs are too heavy to move, and a long-standing pattern of sensitivity to perceived interpersonal rejection

B

behavioral rehearsal—rehearsing new responses to problematic situations

C

catatonic features—clinical features characterized by marked psychomotor disturbance that may involve immobility, excessive motor activity, extreme negativism, inability or refusal to speak, peculiar voluntary movements or speech

circadian rhythms—the daily regulation of sleep-wake cycles and activity-to-activity patterns

cotransmitters—two molecules released from the same synapse that act on an adjacent neuron, both of which are physiologically active

crossover design—a type of clinical study where patients are randomized to one treatment arm, then at some point during the study will be "crossed over" to receive the other treatment option

D

delusions—false, fixed, odd, or unusual beliefs about external reality that are not accepted by other members of the person's culture or subculture yet are firmly sustained despite clear evidence to the contrary

depression—a mood state characterized by sadness or irritability, low energy, thoughts of death and suicide, and lack of interest in previously enjoyed activities

derailment—quality of speech characterized by loose associations or an inability to stay on topic; sequential connection between ideas; which are difficult or impossible to follow because the person wanders to relatively or totally unrelated subjects

dopamine—a neurotransmitter in the central nervous system that affects the synthesis of epinephrine

E

embolic stroke—a type of ischemic stroke that occurs when a blood clot or a cholesterol plaque travels into the brain and blocks an artery

euthymia—normal range of mood, no evidence of mania, hypomania, or depression

evidence-based studies—information about the effectiveness of a treatment gained through rigorously designed, placebo-controlled, double-blind studies

executive functions—those functions of the brain carried out by the prefrontal and frontal cortex: managing stimuli, marshaling appropriate responses, and modulating impulses, which are all disrupted in the manic state

extrapyramidal symptoms—Parkinson-like side effects, such as flat facial expression, stiff muscles, and slowed movements

G

goal-directed behavior—behavior directed towards accomplishing a specific task(s)

grandiosity—exaggerated belief or claims of one's importance or identity; manifested as delusions of great wealth, power, or fame when of psychotic proportions

H

hallucinations—sensory perceptions (seeing, hearing, feeling, and smelling) in the absence of an outside stimulus

hippocampus—an important part of the limbic system involved in working memory and other functions

hormone receptors—a group of molecules that have diverse function throughout the brain and the body (e.g., steroid or estrogen receptors)

hypomania—a mood state characterized by increased energy, excitement, and feelings of euphoria that do not meet the diagnostic criteria for a full manic episode

I

impulsivity—taking action with limited thought to consequences

insight—understanding or awareness of one's mental or emotional condition

interitem reliability—degree to which scores on individual items agree with each other; an estimate of the extent to which the instrument is measuring a single construct.

interrater reliability—degree that different raters agree on a diagnosis based on the use of the instrument

M

maintenance treatment—an ongoing treatment believed to prevent or minimize the development of new episodes of mania, depression, or mixed states

major neurochemical receptor groups—neurotransmitter substances believed important in the normal and abnormal brain functioning

mania—a mood state characterized by an elevated or irritable mood, decreased sleep, high energy, impulsive behavior, and increased goal-directed behavior

melancholic features—loss of interest or pleasure in all, or almost all activities, and lack of reactivity to usually pleasurable stimuli

mixed episodes—periods during which criteria for both a manic and depressive episode are met during the same period of time.

mixed hypomania—this term describes those individuals who meet the criteria for hypomania, but also experience simultaneous symptoms of dysphoria and depression that do not meet the full criteria for a depressive episode

N

neuropeptides—brain chemicals or medications that either decrease cell death and/or increase the birth of new brain cells (i.e., neurogenesis)

neuroprotective effect—the function of a brain chemical or medication to either decrease cell death and/or increase the birth of new brain cells (i.e., neurogenesis)

neurotransmitter—a chemical in the brain that transmits information between the nerve cells

neurotrophins—a class of molecules that triggers changes in the second messenger system(s), increasing cell survival and new cell growth

P

paranormal phenomena—altered perceptions experienced by the patient but not those around him or her (e.g., auditory hallucinations (hearing voices), olfactory hallucinations (smelling burning rubber), and also déjà vu (the sense of having already experienced what is now happening).

PET imaging—technology that uses positron-labeled molecules and an oxygen blood flow tracer to develop images of brain activity versus the structural images provided by MRI

prodromal—precursor to a full episode, or less than criteria for a full-blown episode; subsyndromal symptoms

psychoeducation—teaching patients and/or family members about the illness, treatments, and relapse prevention

psychosis—extreme impairment of a person's ability to think clearly, perceive things accurately, respond emotionally, communicate effectively, understand reality, and behave appropriately

R

rapid cycling—four or more manic, hypomanic, or depressive episodes in any 12-month period

rate of initial titration—the rate by which a medication is increased to what is believed to be a minimum effective dose

role-playing—learning new communication skills by acting out conversations in therapeutic sessions

S

seasonal pattern—onset and remission of depressive symptoms occur at characteristic times of the year

second-generation antipsychotics—the class of antipsychotic medications with fewer extrapyramidal side effects; although the medications in this class share this benefit, they have very different mechanisms of action

sensitivity—the degree to which the instrument correctly identifies patients that do have the disorder

serotonin—a neurotransmitter from the indoleamine group that affects central nervous system functioning

somatization—multiple physical complaints involving any body system

specificity—the degree to which the instrument correctly identifies patients that do not have the disorder

specifiers—DSM-IV-defined categories for specific symptoms that may occur with bipolar disorder, such as psychotic or atypical symptoms

SPECT imaging—a single photon emission where image intensity is directly correlated to cerebral perfusion or blood flow, which is believed to be related to brain functional activity

T

T-scores—standardized scores based on 0 to 100, with 50 as a mean

tangentiality—speech characterized by giving unrelated answers to direct questions and frequently changing the topic

tardive dyskinesia—development of involuntary motor movements, which may persist beyond use of the medication, usually associated with first-generation antipsychotics

temporal lobe—a large lobe of each cerebral hemisphere that is in front of the occipital lobe and is believed involved in memory, mood regulation, and impulsivity

V

vagal nerve stimulation—an FDA-approved treatment for refractory epilepsy and depression now being explored for bipolar disorder

References

Akiskal, H. S. (1996). The prevalent clinical spectrum of bipolar disorders: Beyond DSM-IV. *Journal of Clinical Psychopharmacology, 16*(Suppl. 1), 4S–14S.

Altman, E. G., Hedeker, D., Peterson, J. L., & Davis, J. M. (1997). The Altman Self-Rating Mania Scale. *Biological Psychiatry, 42,* 948–955.

Altman, E. G., Hedeker, D. R., Janicak, P. G., Peterson, J. L., & Davis, J. M. (1994). The Clinician-Administered Rating Scale for Mania (CARS-M): Development, reliability, and validity. *Biological Psychiatry, 36*(2), 124–134.

Altshuler, L., Suppes, T., Black, D., Nolen, W. A., Keck, P. E. Jr., Frye, M. A., et al. (2003). Impact of antidepressant discontinuation after acute bipolar depression remission on rates of depressive relapse at 1-year follow-up. *American Journal of Psychiatry, 160*(7), 1252–1262.

American Diabetes Association, American Psychiatric Association, American Association of Clinical Endocrinologists, North American Association for the Study of Obesity. (2004). Consensus development conference on antipsychotic drugs and obesity and diabetes. *Diabetes Care, 27*(2), 596–601.

American Psychiatric Association. (1952). *Diagnostic and statistical manual: Mental disorders.* Washington, DC: Author.

American Psychiatric Association. (2000). *Diagnostic and statistical manual of mental disorders* (4th ed., text rev.). Washington, DC: Author.

Angst, J., Gamma, A., Benazzi, F., Ajdacic, V., Eich, D., & Rossler, W. (2003). Toward a re-definition of subthreshold bipolarity: Epidemiology and proposed criteria for bipolar-II, minor bipolar disorders and hypomania. *Journal of Affective Disorders, 73*(1–2), 133–146.

Baldessarini, R. J., & Tondo, L. (2008). Lithium and suicidal risk. *Bipolar Disorders, 10,* 114–115.

Baldessarini, R. J., Tondo, L., & Hennen, J. (2003). Lithium treatment and suicide risk in major affective disorders: Update and new findings. *Journal of Clinical Psychiatry, 64*(Suppl. 5), 44–52.

Ball, J. R., Mitchell, P. B., Corry, J. C., Skillicorn, A., Smith, M., & Mahli, G. S. (2006). A randomized controlled trial of cognitive therapy for bipolar disorder; focus on long-term change. *Journal of Clinical Psychiatry, 67,* 277–286.

Basco, M. R., & Rush, A. J. (2005). *Cognitive-behavioral therapy for Bipolar Disorder* (2nd ed.). New York: Guilford Press.

Bauer, M., & Dopfmer, S. (1999). Lithium augmentation in treatment-resistant depression: Meta-analysis of placebo-controlled studies. *Journal of Clinical Psychopharmacology, 19*(5), 427–434.

Bauer, M., & McBride, L. (1996). *Structured group psychotherapy for bipolar disorder: The Life Goals Program.* New York: Springer.

Bauer, M. S., Crits-Christoph, P., Ball, W. A., Dewees, E., McAllister, T., Alahi, P., et al. (1991). Independent assessment of manic and depressive symptoms by self-rating: scale characteristics and implications for the study of mania. *Archives of General Psychiatry, 48*(9), 807–812.

Bauer, M. S., Kirk, G. F., Gavin, C., & Williford, W. O. (2001). Determinants of functional outcome and healthcare costs in bipolar disorder: A high-intensity follow-up study. *Journal of Affective Disorders, 65*(3), 231–241.

Bauer, M. S., McBride, L., Williford, W. O., Glick, H., Kinosian, B., Altshuler, L., et al. (2006a). Collaborative care for bipolar disorder: Part I. Intervention and implementation in a randomized effectiveness trial. *Psychiatric Services, 57*(7), 927–936.

Bauer, M. S., McBride, L., Williford, W. O., Glick, H., Kinosian, B., Altshuler, L., et al. (2006b). Collaborative care for bipolar disorder: Part II. Impact on clinical outcome, function, and costs. *Psychiatric Services, 57*(7), 937–945.

Beck, A. T., Brown, G., Berchick, R. J., Stewart, B. L., & Steer, R. A. (1990). Relationship between hopelessness and ultimate suicide: A replication with psychiatric outpatients. *American Journal of Psychiatry, 147*(2), 190–195.

Beck, A. T., Steer, R. A., & Brown, G. K. (1986). *Beck Depression Inventory-Second Edition Manual.* San Antonio, TX: Psychological Corporation, Harcourt Brace.

Beck, A. T., Steer, R. A., & Garbin, M. G. (1988). Psychometric properties of the Beck Depression Inventory: Twenty-five years of evaluation. *Clinical Psychology Review, 8,* 77–100.

Beck, A. T., Steer, R. A., Kovacs, M., & Garrison, B. (1985). Hopelessness and eventual suicide: A 10-year prospective study of patients hospitalized with suicidal ideation. *American Journal of Psychiatry, 142*(5), 559–563.

Belmaker, R. H. (2007). Treatment of bipolar depression. *New England Journal of Medicine, 356,* 1771–1773.

Benazzi, F. (2000). Depression with DSM-IV atypical features: A marker for Bipolar II disorder. *European Archives of Psychiatry and Clinical Neuroscience, 250,* 53–55.

Benazzi, F. (2007). Testing a new diagnostic criteria for hypomania. *Annals of Clinical Psychiatry, 19,* 1–6.

Berk, M., Ichim, L., & Brook, S. (1999). Olanzapine compared to lithium in mania: A double-blind randomized controlled trial. *International Clinical Psychopharmacology, 14*(6), 339–343.

Bigelow, L., & Murphy, D. L. (1978). *Guidelines and anchor points for modified BPRS.* Unpublished manuscript, NIMH Intramural Research Program, Saint Elizabeth's Hospital.

Boerlin, H. L., Gitlin, M. J., Zoellner, L. A., Hammen, C. L., et al. (1998). Bipolar depression and antidepressant-induced mania: A naturalistic study. *Journal of Clinical Psychiatry, 59*(7), 374–379.

Bowden, C. L. (2001). Strategies to reduce misdiagnosis of bipolar depression. *Psychiatric Services, 52*(1), 51–55.

Bowden, C. L., Brugger, A. M., Swann, A. C, Calabrese, J. R., Janicak, P. G., Petty, F., et al. (1994). Efficacy of divalproex vs lithium and placebo in the treatment of mania. The Depakote Mania Study Group. *Journal of the American Medical Association, 271*(12), 918–924.

Bowden, C. L., Calabrese, J. R., McElroy, S. L., Gyulai, L., Wassef, A., Petty, F. et al. (2000). A randomized, placebo-controlled 12-month trial of divalproex and lithium in treatment of outpatients with bipolar I disorder. *Archives of General Psychiatry, 57,* 481–489.

Bowden, C. L., Calabrese, J. R., Sachs, G., Yatham, L. N., Asghar, S. A., Hompland, M., et al. (2003). A placebo-controlled 18-month trial of lamotrigine and lithium maintenance treatment in recently manic or hypomanic patients with bipolar I disorder. *Archives of General Psychiatry, 60*(4), 392–400.

Bowden, C. L., Grunze, H., Mullen, J., Brecher, M., Paulsson, B., Jones, M., et al. (2005). A randomized, double-blind, placebo-controlled efficacy and safety study of quetiapine or lithium as monotherapy for mania in bipolar disorder. *Journal of Clinical Psychiatry, 66*(1), 111–121.

Bowden, C. L., Vieta, E., Ice, K. S., Schwartz, J. H., Wang, P. P., & Versavel, M. (2010). Ziprasidone plus a mood stabilizer in subjects with bipolar I disorder: A 6-month, randomized, placebo-controlled, double-blind trial. *Journal of Clinical Psychiatry, 71*(2), 130–137.

Brown, E. B., McElroy, S. L., Keck, P. E., Jr., Deldar, A., Adams, D. H., Tohen, M., et al. (2006). A 7-week, randomized, double-blind trial of olanzapine/fluoxetine combination versus lamotrigine in the treatment of bipolar I depression. *Journal of Clinical Psychiatry, 67,* 1025–1033.

Butcher, J. N., Dahlstrom, W. G., Graham, J. R., Tellegen, A., & Kaemmer, B. (1989). *Minnesota Multiphasic Personality Inventory-2 (MMPI-2): Manual for Administration and Scoring.* Minneapolis, MN: University of Minnesota Press.

Cade, J. F. J. (1949). Lithium salts in the treatment of psychotic excitement. *Medical Journal of Australia, 36,* 349–352.

Calabrese, J. R., Bowden, C. L., Sachs, G., Yatham, L. N., Behnke, K., Mehtonen, O., et al. (2003). A placebo-controlled 18-month trial of lamotrigine and lithium maintenance treatment in recently depressed patients with bipolar I disorder. *Journal of Clinical Psychiatry, 64,* 1013–1024.

Calabrese, J. R., Huffman, R. F., White, R. L., Edwards, S., Thompson, T. R., Ascher, J. A., et al. (2008). Lamotrigine in the acute treatment of bipolar depression: Results of five double-blind, placebo-controlled clinical trials. *Bipolar Disorders, 10,* 323–333.

Calabrese, J. R., Kimmel, S. E., Woyshville, M. J, Rapport, D. J., Faust, C. J., Thompson, P. A., et al. (1996). Clozapine for treatment-refractory mania. *American Journal of Psychiatry, 153,* 759–764.

Calabrese, J. R., Shelton, M. D., Rapport, D. J., Youngstrom, E. A., Jackson, K., Bilali, S., et al. (2005). A 20-month, double-blind, maintenance trial of lithium versus divalproex in rapid-cycling bipolar disorder. *American Journal of Psychiatry, 162,* 2152–2161.

Carlson, G. A. (1998). Mania and ADHD: Comorbidity or confusion. *Journal of Affective Disorders, 51*(2), 177–187.

Cassano, G. B., Frank, E., Miniati, M., Rucci, P., Fagiolini, A., Pini, S., et al. (2002). Conceptual underpinnings and empirical support for the mood spectrum. *Psychiatric Clinics of North America, 25*(4), 699–712.

Citrome, L. L., & Jaffe, A. B. (2003). Relationship of atypical antipsychotics with development of diabetes mellitus. *Annals of Pharmacotherapy, 37*(12), 1849–1857.

Cochran, S. (1984). Preventing medical noncompliance in the outpatient treatment of bipolar affective disorders. *Journal of Consulting and Clinical Psychology, 52,* 873–878.

Cohn, J. B., Collins, G., Ashbrook, E., & Wernicke, J. F. (1989). A comparison of fluoxetine imipramine and placebo in patients with bipolar depressive disorder. *International Clinical Psychopharmacology, 4*(4), 313–322.

Colom, F., & Vieta, E. (2006). *Psychoeducation manual for bipolar disorder.* Cambridge University Press.

Colom, F., Vieta, E., Martinez-Aran, A., Reinares, M., Goikolea, J. M., Benabarre, A., et al. (2003). A randomized trial on the efficacy of group psychoeducation in the prophylaxis of recurrences in bipolar patients whose disease is in remission. *Archives of General Psychiatry, 60,* 402–407.

Colom, F., Vieta, E., Reinares, M., Martínez-Arán, A., Torrent, C., Goikolea, J. M., et al. (2003). Psychoeducation efficacy in bipolar disorders: Beyond compliance enhancement. *Journal of Clinical Psychiatry, 64*(9), 1101–1105.

Colom, F., Vieta, E., Tacchi, M. J., Sanchez-Moreno, J., & Scott, J. (2005a). Identifying and improving non-adherence in bipolar disorders. *Bipolar Disorders, 7,* 24–31.

Colom, F., Vieta, E., Sanchez-Moreno, J., Martínez-Arán, A., Reinares, M., Goikolea, J. M., et al. (2005b). Stabilizing the stabilizer: Group psychoeducation enhances the stability of serum lithium levels. *Bipolar Disorders, 7*(Suppl. 5), 32–36.

Coryell, W., Scheftner, W., Keller, M., Endicott, J., Maser, J., & Klerman, G. L. (1993). The enduring psychosocial consequences of mania and depression. *American Journal of Psychiatry, 150,* 720–727.

Davidson, J., Turnbull, C. D., Strickland, R., Miller, R., & Graves, K. (1986). The Montgomery-Äsberg Depression Scale: Reliability and validity. *Acta Psychiatrica Scandinavica, 73,* 544–548.

Davis, L. L., Bartolucci, A., & Petty, F. (2005). Divalproex in the treatment of bipolar depression: A placebo-controlled study. *Journal of Affective Disorders, 85,* 259–266.

Denicoff, K. D., Leverich, G. S., Nolen, W. A., Rush, A. J., McElroy, S. L., Keck, P. E. Jr., et al. (2000). Validation of the prospective NIMH-Life-Chart Method (NIMH-LCM™-p) for longitudinal assessment of Bipolar illness. *Psychological Medicine, 30,* 1391–1397.

Dennehy, E. B., Schnyer, R., Bernstein, I. H., Gonzalez, R., Shivakumar, G., Kelly, D. I., et al. (2009). The safety, acceptability, and effectiveness of acupuncture as an adjunctive treatment for bipolar disorder. *Journal of Clinical Psychiatry, 70*(6), 897–905. Epub May 5, 2009 (doi 10.4088.JCP.08m04208).

Department of Veterans Affairs/Department of Defense. (2010). Management of Bipolar Disorder in adults (BD). http://www.healthquality.va.gov/Management_of_Bi.asp, accessed August 5, 2010.

Dion, G., Tohen, M., Anthony, W., & Waternaux, C. (1988). Symptoms and functioning of patients with Bipolar Disorder six months after hospitalization. *Hospital & Community Psychiatry, 39,* 652–656.

Ebert, D., Jaspert, A., Murata, H., & Kaschka, W. P. (1995). Initial lithium augmentation improves the antidepressant effects of standard TCA treatment in non-resistant depressed patients. *Psychopharmacology, 118*(2), 223–225.

Endicott, J., & Spitzer, R. L. (1978). A diagnostic interview: The schedule for affective disorders and schizophrenia. *Archives of General Psychiatry, 35*(7), 837–844.

Ernst, C. L., & Goldberg, J. F. (2004). Antisuicide properties of psychotropic drugs: A critical review. *Harvard Review of Psychiatry, 12,* 14–41.

Ernst, E. (2002). Safety concerns about kava. *Lancet. 359,* 1865.

Essock, S. M., Hargreaves, W. A., Covell, N. H., & Goethe, J. (1996). Clozapine's effectiveness for patients in state hospitals: Results from a randomized trial. *Psychopharmacology Bulletin, 32*(4), 683–697.

Faraone, S. V., Glatt, S. J., & Tsuang, M. T. (2003). The genetics of pediatric-onset Bipolar Disorder. *Biological Psychiatry. 53,* 970–977.

Faraone, S. V., & Tsuang, M. T. (2003). Heterogeneity and the genetics of Bipolar Disorder. *American Journal of Medical Genetics, 123C,* 1–9.

Fieve, R. R., Kumbaraci, T., & Dunner, D. L. (1976). Lithium prophylaxis of depression in bipolar I, bipolar II, and unipolar patients. *American Journal of Psychiatry, 133*(8), 925–929.

First, M. B., Spitzer, R. L., Gibbon, M., & Williams, J. B. W. (1997). *Structured Clinical Interview for DSM-IV-Clinician Version (SCID-CV) (User's Guide and Interview).* Washington, DC: American Psychiatric Press.

Frank, E., Hlastala, S., Ritenour, A., Houck, P., Tu, X. M., Monk, T. H., et al. (1997). Inducing lifestyle regularity in recovering Bipolar Disorder patients: Results from the maintenance therapies in Bipolar Disorder protocol. *Biological Psychiatry, 41,* 1165–1173.

Frank, E., Kupfer, D. J., Thase, M. E., Mallinger, A. G., Swartz, H. A., Fagiolini, A. M., et al. (2005). Two-year outcomes for interpersonal and social rhythm therapy in individuals with bipolar I disorder. *Archives of General Psychiatry, 62*(9), 996–1004.

Frank, E., Swartz, H. A., & Kupfer, D. J. (2000). Interpersonal and social rhythm therapy: Managing the chaos of Bipolar Disorder. *Biological Psychiatry, 48*(6), 593–604.

Frye, M. A., Altshuler, L. L., McElroy, S. L., Suppes, T., Keck, P. E., Denicoff, K., et al. (2003). Gender differences in prevalence, risk, and clinical correlates of alcoholism comorbidity in bipolar disorder. *American Journal of Psychiatry, 160*(5), 883–889.

Frye, M. A., Ketter, T. A., Altshuler, L. L., Denicoff, K., Dunn, R. T., Kimbrell, T. A., et al. (1998). Clozapine in Bipolar Disorder: treatment implications for other atypical antipsychotics. *Journal of Affective Disorders, 48*(2–3), 91–104.

Geddes, J. R., Burgess, S., Hawton, K., Jamison, K., & Goodwin, G. M. (2004). Long-term lithium therapy for bipolar disorder: Systematic review and meta-analysis of randomized controlled trials. *American Journal of Psychiatry, 161,* 217–222.

Geddes, J. R., Calabrese, J. R., & Goodwin, G. M. (2009). Lamotrigine for treatment of bipolar depression: An independence meta-analysis and meta-regression of individual patient data from 5 randomized controlled trials. *British Journal of Psychiatry, 194,* 4–9.

Ghaemi, S. N., Berv, D. A., Klugman, J., Rosenquist, K. J., & Hsu, D. J. (2003). Oxcarbazepine treatment of Bipolar Disorder. *Journal of Clinical Psychiatry, 64,* 943–945.

Ghaemi, S. N., Gilmer, W. S., Goldberg, J. F., Zablotsky, B., Kemp, D. E., Kelley, M. E., et al. (2007). Divalproex in the treatment of acute bipolar depression: A preliminary double-blind, randomized, placebo-controlled pilot study. *Journal of Clinical Psychiatry, 68,* 1840–1844.

Gijsman, H. J., Geddes, J. R., Rendell, J. M., Nolen, W. A., Goodwin, G. M. (2004). Antidepressants for bipolar depression: A systematic review of randomized, controlled trials. *American Journal of Psychiatry, 161,* 1537–1547.

Goldberg, J. F., Burdick, K. E., & Endick, C. J. (2004). Preliminary randomized, double-blind, placebo-controlled trial of pramipexole added to mood stabilizers for treatment-resistant bipolar depression. *American Journal of Psychiatry, 161,* 564–566.

Goldberg, J. F., Garno, J. L., Leon, A. C., Kocsis, J. H., Portera, L. (1999). A history of substance abuse complicates remission from acute mania in bipolar disorder. *Journal of Clinical Psychiatry, 60*(11), 733–740.

Gonzalez-Pinto, A., Gonzalez, C., Enjuto, S., Fernandez de Corres, B., Lopez, L., Palomo, J., et al. (2004). Psychoeducation and cognitive-behavioral therapy in bipolar disorder: An update. *Acta Psychiatrica Scandinavica, 109*(2), 83–90.

Goodwin, F. K., & Jamison, K. R. (2007). *Manic-depressive illness: Bipolar disorders and recurrent depression* (2nd ed.). New York: Oxford University Press.

Goodwin, G. M., Bowden, C. L., Calabrese, J. R., Grunze, H., Kasper, S., White, R. et al. (2004). A pooled analysis of 2 placebo-controlled 18-month trials of lamotrigine and lithium maintenance in bipolar I disorder. *Journal of Clinical Psychiatry, 65,* 432–441.

Grunze, H. (2003). Lithium in the acute treatment of Bipolar Disorders—a stocktaking. *European Archives of Psychiatry and Clinical Neuroscience, 253,* 115–119.

Hamilton, M. (1960). A rating scale for depression. *Journal of Neurology, Neurosurgery, and Psychiatry, 23,* 56–62.

Hamilton, M. (1967). Development of a rating scale for primary depressive illness. *British Journal of Social and Clinical Psychology, 6,* 278–296.

Hayden, E. P., & Nurnberger, J. I., Jr. (2006). Molecular genetics of bipolar disorder. *Genes, Brain, and Behavior, 5,* 85–95.

Helzer, J. E., Spitznagel, E. L., & McEvoy, L. (1987). The predictive validity of lay Diagnostic Interview Schedule diagnoses in the general population. A comparison with physician examiners. *Archives of General Psychiatry, 44*(12), 1069–1077.

Himmelhoch, J. M., Thase, M. E., Mallinger, A. G., & Houck, P. (1991). Tranylcypromine versus imipramine in anergic bipolar depression. *American Journal of Psychiatry, 148*(7), 910–916.

Hirschfeld, R., and Compact Clinicals. (2005). Mood Disorder Questionnaire–Expanded. Kansas City, MO: Compact Clinicals.

Hirschfeld, R. M., Holzer, C., Calabrese, J. R., Weissman, M., Reed, M., Davies, M., et al. (2003). Validity of the mood disorder questionnaire: A general population study. *American Journal of Psychiatry, 160,* 178–180.

Hirschfeld, R. M., Holzer, C., Calabrese, J. R., Weissman, M., Reed, M., Davies, M., et al. (2003). Validity of the mood disorder questionnaire: A general population study. *American Journal of Psychiatry, 160,* 178–180.

Hirschfeld, R. M., Keck, P. E., Jr., Kramer, M., Karcher, K., Canuso, C., Eerdekens, M., et al. (2004). Rapid antimanic effect of risperidone monotherapy: A 3-week multicenter, double-blind, placebo-controlled trial. *American Journal of Psychiatry, 161*(6), 1057–1065.

Hirschfeld, R. M. A., Bowden, D. L., Gitlin, M. J., Keck, P. E., Perlis, R. H., Suppes, T., et al. (2002). Practice Guideline for the treatment of patients with Bipolar Disorder (revision). *American Journal of Psychiatry, 159* (Suppl.), 1–50.

Hirschfeld, R. M. A., Williams, J. B. W., Spitzer, R. L., Calabrese, J. R., Flynn, L., Keck, P. E. Jr., et al. (2000). Development and validation of a screening instrument for Bipolar spectrum disorder: the Mood Disorder Questionnaire. *American Journal of Psychiatry, 157,* 1873–1875.

Isojarvi, J. I., Laatikainen, T. J., Pakarinen, A. J., Juntunen, K. T., & Myllyla, V. V. (1993). Polycystic ovaries and hyperandrogenism in women taking valproate for epilepsy. *New England Journal of Medicine, 329,* 1383–1388.

Joffe, H., Cohen, L. S., Suppes, T., McLaughlin, W. L., Lavori, P., Adams, J. M., et al. (2006). Valproate is associated with new-onset oligoamenorrhea with hyperandrogenism in women with bipolar disorder. *Biological Psychiatry. 59*(11), 1078–1086.

Johnson, S. L., & Roberts, J. E. (1995). Life events and Bipolar Disorder: Implications from biological theories. *Psychological Bulletin, 117,* 434–449.

Johnson, S. L., Winett, C. A., Meyer, B., Greenhouse, W. J., & Miller, I. (1999). Social support and the course of Bipolar Disorder. *Journal of Abnormal Psychology,* 108, 558–566.

Judd, L. L., Akiskal, H. S., Schettler, P. J., Endicott, J., Leon, A. C., Solomon, D. A., et al. (2005). Psychosocial disability in the course of bipolar I and II disorders: A prospective, comparative, longitudinal study. *Archives of General Psychiatry, 62*(12), 1322–1330.

Kearns, N. P., Cruickshank, C. A., McGuigan, K. J., Riley, S. A., Shaw, S. P., & Snaith, R. P. (1982). A comparison of depression rating scales. *British Journal of Psychiatry, 141,* 45–49.

Keck, P. E., Jr., Calabrese, J. R., McIntyre, R. S., McQuade, R. D., Carson, W. H., Eudicone, J. M., et al. (2007). Aripiprazole monotherapy for maintenance therapy in bipolar I disorder: A 100-week, double blind study versus placebo. *Journal of Clinical Psychiatry, 68,* 1480–1491.

Keck, P. E., Jr., Calabrese, J. R., McQuade, R. D., Carson, W. H., Carlson, B. X., Rollin, L. M., et al. (2006). A randomized, double-blind, placebo-controlled 26-week trial of aripiprazole in recently manic patients with bipolar I disorder. *Journal of Clinical Psychiatry, 67,* 626–637.

Keck P. E, Jr., Marcus, R., Tourkodimitris, S., Ali, M., Liebeskind, A., Saha, A., et al. (2003). A placebo-controlled, double-blind study of the efficacy and safety of aripiprazole in patients with acute bipolar mania. *American Journal of Psychiatry, 160,* 1651–1658.

Keck, P. E. Jr., Perlis, R. H., Otto, M. W., Carpenter, D., Ross, R., Docherty, J. P. (2004). The Expert Consensus Guideline Series: Treatment of Bipolar Disorder 2004. *Postgraduate Medicine Special Report,* 1–120.

Keck, P. E., Jr., Versiani, M., Potkin, S., West, S. A., Giller, E., & Ice, K. Ziprasidone in the treatment of acute bipolar mania: A three-week, placebo-controlled, double-blind, randomized trial. *American Journal of Psychiatry, 160*(4), 741–748.

Kessler, R. C., Berguland, P., Demler, O., Jin, R., & Walters, E. E. (2005a). Lifetime prevalence and age-of-onset distributions of DSM-IV disorders in the national comorbidity survey replication. *Archives of General Psychiatry, 62,* 593–602.

Kessler, R. C., Chiu, W. T., Demler, O., Walters, E. E. (2005b). Prevalence, severity, and comorbidity of 12-month DSM-IV disorders in the National Comorbidity Survey Replication. *Archives of General Psychiatry, 62*(6), 617–627.

Ketter, R. A., Kalali, A. H., & Weisler, R. H. (2004). A 6-month, multicenter, open-label evaluation of beaded, extended-release carbamazepine capsule monotherapy in bipolar disorder patients with manic or mixed episodes. *Journal of Clinical Psychiatry, 65,* 668–673.

Ketter, T. A., Post, R. M., Parekh, P. I., & Worthington, K. (1995). Addition of monoamine oxidase inhibitors to carbamazepine: Preliminary evidence of safety and antidepressant efficacy in treatment-resistant depression. *Journal of Clinical Psychiatry, 56*(10), 471–475.

Khanna, S., Vieta, E., Lyons, B., Grossman, F., Eerdekens, M., & Kramer, M. (2005). Risperidone in the treatment of acute mania: Double-blind, placebo-controlled study. *British Journal of Psychiatry, 187,* 229–234.

Klerman, G. L., Weissman, M. M., Rounsaville, B. J., & Chevron, R. S. (1984). *Interpersonal psychotherapy of depression.* New York: Basic Books.

Kowatch, R. A., Fristad, M., Birmaher, B., Wagner, K. D., Findling, R. L., Hellander, M., Child Psychiatric Workgroup on Bipolar Disorder. (2005). Treatment guidelines for children and adolescents with bipolar disorder. *Journal of the American Academy of Child and Adolescent Psychiatry, 44*(3), 213–235.

Kupfer, D. J., Chengappa, K. N., Gelenberg, A. J., Hirschfeld, R. M. A., Goldberg, J. F., et al. (2001). Citalopram as adjunctive therapy in bipolar depression. *Journal of Clinical Psychiatry, 62*(12), 985–990.

Kupka, R. W., Luckenbaugh, D.A., Post, R. M., Leverich, G. S., & Nolen, W. A. (2003). Rapid and non-rapid cycling bipolar disorder: A meta-analysis of clinical studies. *Journal of Clinical Psychiatry, 64,* 1483–1494.

Kupka, R. W., Luckenbaugh, D. A., Post, R. M., Suppes, T., Altshuler, L. L., Keck, P. E. Jr., et al. (2005). Comparison of rapid-cycling and non-rapid-cycling bipolar disorder based on prospective mood ratings in 539 outpatients. *American Journal of Psychiatry, 162,* 1273–1280.

Lam, D. H., Hayward P., Watkins, E. R., Wright, K., & Sham, P. (2005). Relapse prevention in patients with bipolar disorder: Cognitive therapy outcome after 2 years. *American Journal of Psychiatry, 162,* 324–329.

Lam, D. H., Watkins, E. R., Hayward, P., Bright, J., Wright, K., Kerr, N., et al. (2003). A randomized controlled study of cognitive therapy for relapse prevention for bipolar affective disorder. *Archives of General Psychiatry, 60,* 145–152.

Leverich, G. S., Altshuler, L. L., Frye, M. A., Suppes, T., McElroy, S. L., Keck, P. E. Jr., et al. (2006). Risk of switch in mood polarity to hypomania or mania in patients with bipolar depression during acute and continuation trials of venlafaxine, sertraline, and bupropion as adjuncts to mood stabilizers. *American Journal of Psychiatry, 163*(2), 232–239.

Leverich, G. S., & Post, R. M. (1998). Life charting of affective disorders. *CNS Spectrums, 3*(5), 21–37.

Lingam, R., & Scott, J. (2002). Treatment non-adherence in affective disorders. *Acta Psychiatrica Scandinavica, 105*(3), 164–72.

Macfadden, W., Alphs, L., Haskins, J. T., Turner, N., Turkoz, I., Bossie, C., et al. (2009). A randomized, double-blind, placebo-controlled study of maintenance treatment with adjunctive risperidone long-acting therapy in patients with bipolar I disorder who relapse frequently. *Bipolar Disorders, 11,* 827–839. doi: 10.1111/j.1399-5618.2009.00761.x

MacQueen, G. M., Young, L. T., & Joffe, R. T. (2001). A review of psychosocial outcome in patients with bipolar disorder. *Acta Psychiatrica Scandinavica, 103*(3), 163–170.

Malkoff-Schwartz, S., Frank, E., Anderson, B. P., Hlastala, S. A., Luther, J. F., Sherrill, J. T., et al. (2000). Social rhythm disruption and stressful life events in the onset of bipolar and unipolar episodes. *Psychological Medicine, 30,* 1005–1016.

Manji, H. K., Moore, G. J., & Chen, G. (2000). Lithium up-regulates the cytoprotective protein Bcl-2 in the CNS in vivo: A role for neurotrophic and neuroprotective effects in manic depressive illness. *Journal of Clinical Psychiatry, 61*(Suppl. 9), 82–96.

Marangell, L. B., Suppes, T., Ketter, T. A., Dennehy, E. B., Zboyan, H., Kertz, B., et al. (2006). Omega-3 fatty acids in bipolar disorder: Clinical and research considerations. *Prostaglandins, Leukotrienes & Essential Fatty Acids, 75*(4–5), 315–321.

Marangell, L. B., Suppes, T., Zboyan, H. A., Prashad, S. J., Fischer, G., Snow, D., et al. (2008). A 1-year pilot study of vagus nerve stimulation in treatment-resistant rapid-cycling bipolar disorder. *Journal of Clinical Psychiatry, 69,* 183–189.

McClellan, J., Kowatch, R., & Findling, R. L. (2007). Practice parameter for the assessment and treatment of children and adolescents with bipolar disorder. *Journal of the American Academy of Child & Adolescent Psychiatry, 46,* 107–125.

McElroy, S., Altshuler, L., Suppes, T., Keck, P. E. Jr., Frye, M. A., Denicoff, K. D., et al. (2001). Axis I psychiatric comorbidity and its relationship to historical illness variables in 288 patients with bipolar disorder. *American Journal of Psychiatry, 158,* 3.

McElroy, S. L., Bowden, C. L., Collins, M. A., Wozniak, P. J., Keck, P. E., Jr., & Calabrese, J. R. (2008). Relationship of open acute mania treatment to blinded maintenance outcome in bipolar I disorder. *Journal of Affective Disorders, 107,* 127–133.

McElroy, S. L., Dessain, E. C., Pope, H. G., Jr., Cole, J. O., Keck, P. E. Jr., Frankenberg, F. R., et al. (1991). Clozapine in the treatment of psychotic mood disorders, schizoaffective disorder, and schizophrenia. *Journal of Clinical Psychiatry, 52*(10), 411–414.

McElroy, S. L., Weisler, R. H., Chang, W., Olausson, B., Paulsson, B., Brecher, M., Agambaram, V., et al. (2010). A double-blind, placebo-controlled study of quetiapine and paroxetine as monotherapy in adults with bipolar depression (EMBOLDEN II). *Journal of Clinical Psychiatry, 71*(2), 163–174.

McIntyre, R., Brecher, M., Poulsson, B., Huizar, K., & Mullen, J. (2005). Quetiapine or haloperidol as monotherapy for bipolar mania—a 12-week, double-blind, randomised, parallel-group, placebo-controlled trial. *European Neuropsychopharmacology, 15,* 573–585.

McIntyre, R., Hirschfeld, R., Alphs, L., Cohen, M., Macek, T., & Panagides, J. (2008). Asenapine in the treatment of acute mania in bipolar I disorder: Outcomes from two randomized placebo-controlled trials. *Bipolar Disorders, 10*(Suppl. 1), 49.

McIntyre, R. S., Cohen, M., Zhao, J., Alphs, L., Macek, T. A., & Panagides, J. (2009a). A 3-week, randomized, placebo-controlled trial of asenapine in the treatment of acute mania in bipolar mania and mixed states. *Bipolar Disorders, 11,* 673–686.

McIntyre, R. S., Cohen, M., Zhao, J., Alphs, L., Macek, T. A., & Panagides, J. (2009b). Asenapine versus olanzapine in acute mania: A double-blind extension study. *Bipolar Disorders, 11,* 815–826.

Merikangas, K. R., Akiskal, H. S., Angst, J., Greenberg, P. E., Hirschfeld, R. M., Petukhova, M., et al. (2007). Lifetime and 12-month prevalence of bipolar spectrum disorder in the National Comorbidity Survey replication. *Archives of General Psychiatry, 64,* 543–552.

Miklowitz, D. J. (2008). Adjunctive psychotherapy for bipolar disorder: State of the evidence. *American Journal of Psychiatry, 165*(11), 1408–1419.

Miklowitz, D. J., Axelson, D. A., Birmaher, B., George, E. L., Taylor, D. O., Schneck, C. D., et al. (2008). Family focused treatment for adolescents with bipolar disorder: Results of a 2-year randomized trial. *Archives of General Psychiatry, 65,* 1053–1061.

Miklowitz, D. J., Biuckians, A., Richards, J. A. (2006). Early-onset bipolar disorder: A family treatment perspective. *Development and Psychopathology, 18*(4), 1247–1265.

Miklowitz, D. J., George, E. L., Richards, J. A., Simoneau, T. L., & Suddath, R. L. (2003). A randomized study of family-focused psychoeducation and pharmacotherapy in the outpatient management of bipolar disorder. *Archives of General Psychiatry, 60,* 904–912.

Miklowitz, D. J., & Goldstein, M. J. (1997). *Bipolar disorder: A family-focused treatment approach.* New York: Guilford.

Miklowitz, D. J., Otto, M. W. (2006). New psychosocial interventions for bipolar disorder: A review of literature and introduction of the Systematic Treatment Enhancement Program. *Journal of Cognitive Psychotherapy, 20*(2), 215–230.

Miklowitz, D. J., Otto, M. W., Frank, E., Reilly-Harrington, N. A., Kogan, J. N., Sachs, G. S., et al. (2007). Intensive psychosocial intervention enhances functioning in patients with bipolar depression: Results from a 9-month randomized controlled trial. *American Journal of Psychiatry, 164,* 1340–1347.

Miklowitz, D. J., Richards, J. A., George, E. L., Frank, E., Suddath, R. L., Powell, K. B., et al. (2003). Integrated family and individual therapy for bipolar disorder: Results of a treatment development study. *Journal of Clinical Psychiatry, 64,* 182–191.

Miklowitz, D. J., Simoneau, T. L., & George, E. L. (2000). Family-focused treatment of Bipolar Disorder: 1-year effects of a psychoeducational program in conjunction with pharmacotherapy. *Biological Psychiatry, 4,* 582–592.

Miller, I. W., Keitner, G. I., Ryan, C. E., Uebelacker, L. A., Johnson, S. L., & Solomon, D. A. (2008). Family treatment for bipolar disorder: Family impairment by treatment interactions. *Journal of Clinical Psychiatry, 69*(5), 732–740.

Miller, I. W., Solomon, D. A., Ryan, C. E., & Keitner, G. I. (2004). Does adjunctive family therapy enhance recovery from bipolar I mood episodes? *Journal of Affective Disorders, 82*(3), 431–436.

Millon, T., Davis, R., & Millon, C. (1997). *MCMI-III Manual* (2nd ed.). Minneapolis, MN: National Computer Systems.

Montgomery, S. A., & Äsberg, M. (1979). A new depression scale designed to be sensitive to change. *British Journal of Psychiatry, 134,* 382–389.

Mukherjee, S., Sackeim, H. A., & Schnurr, D. B. (1994). Electroconvulsive therapy of acute manic episode: A review of 50 years' experience. *American Journal of Psychiatry, 151*(2), 169–176.

Murphy, L. L., Impara, J. C., & Plake, B. S. (eds.). (1999). *Tests in print.* V. Lincoln, NE: University of Nebraska Press.

Nemeroff, C. B., Evans, D. L., Gyulai, L., Sachs, G. S., Bowden, C. L., Gergel, I. P., et al. (2001). Double-blind, placebo-controlled comparison of imipramine and paroxetine in the treatment of bipolar depression. *American Journal of Psychiatry. 158,* 906–912.

Otto, M. W., Reilly-Harrington, N., & Sachs, G. S. (2003). Psychoeducational and cognitive-behavioral strategies in the management of bipolar disorder. *Journal of Affective Disorders, 73*(1–2), 171–181.

Overall, J. E., & Gorham, D. R. (1988). Introduction—the Brief Psychiatric Rating Scale (BPRS): Recent developments in ascertainment and scaling. *Psychopharmacology Bulletin, 24,* 97–99.

Padmos, R. C., Van Baal, G. C. M., Vonk, R., Wijkhuijs, A. J. M., Kahn, R. S., Nolen, W. A., et al. (2009). Genetic and environmental influences on pro-inflammatory monocytes in bipolar disorder: A twin study *Archives of General Psychiatry, 66*(9), 957–965. doi:10.1001/archgenpsychiatry.2009.116

Perlick, D. A. (2004). Medication non-adherence in bipolar disorder: A patient-centered review of research findings. *Clinical Approaches in Bipolar Disorders, 3,* 56-64.

Perlis, R. H., Baker, R. W., Zarate, C. A., Jr., Brown, E. B., Schuh, L. M., Jamal, H. H., et al. (2006). Olanzapine versus risperidone in the treatment of manic or mixed states in bipolar I disorder: A randomized, double-blind trial. *Journal of Clinical Psychiatry, 67,* 1747–1753.

Perlis, R. H., Sachs, G. S., Lafer, B., Otto, M. W., Faraone, S. V., Kane, J. M., et al. (2002). Effect of abrupt change from standard to low serum levels of lithium: A reanalysis of double-blind lithium maintenance data. *American Journal of Psychiatry, 159,* 1155–1159.

Perry, A., Tarrier, N., Morriss, R., McCarthy, E., Limb, K. (1999). Randomised controlled trial of efficacy of teaching patients with Bipolar Disorder to identify early symptoms of relapse and obtain treatment. *British Medical Journal, 318,* 149–153.

Pope, H. G., Jr., McElroy, S. L., Keck, P. E., Jr., & Hudson, J. I. (1991). Valproate in the treatment of acute mania. A placebo-controlled study. *Archives of General Psychiatry, 48*(1), 62–68.

Post, R. M., Altshuler, L. L., Frye, M. A., Suppes, T., Rush, A. J., Keck, P. E. Jr., et al. (2001). Rate of switch in bipolar patients prospectively treated with second-generation antidepressants as augmentation to mood stabilizers. *Bipolar Disorders, 3,* 259–265.

Post, R. M., Altshuler, L. L., Leverich, G. S., Frye, M. A., Nolen, W. A., Kupka, R. W., et al. (2006). Mood switch in bipolar depression: Comparison of adjunctive venlafaxine, bupropion and sertraline. *British Journal of Psychiatry, 189,* 124–131.

Post, R. M., Leverich, G. S., Denicoff, K. D., Frye, M. A., Kimbrell, T. A., & Dunn, R. (1997). Alternative approaches to refractory depression in bipolar illness. *Depression and Anxiety, 5*(4), 175–189.

Post, R. M., Leverich, G. S., Nolen, W. A., Kupka, R. W., Altshuler, L. L., Frye, M. A., et al. (2003). A re-evaluation of the role of antidepressants in the treatment of bipolar depression: data from the Stanley Foundation Bipolar Network. *Bipolar Disorders, 5,* 396–406.

Post, R. M., Roy-Byrne, P. P., Uhde, T. W. (1998). Graphic representation of the life course of illness in patients with affective disorder. *American Journal of Psychiatry, 145*(7), 844–848.

Potkin, S. G., Keck, P. E., Jr., Segal, S., Ice, K., & English, P. (2005). Ziprasidone in acute bipolar mania: A 21-day randomized, double-blind, placebo-controlled replication trial. *Journal of Clinical Psychopharmacology, 25,* 301–310.

Potts, M. K., Daniels, M., Burnam, M. A., & Wells, K. B. (1990). A structured interview version of the Hamilton Depression Rating

Scale: Evidence of reliability and versatility of administration. *Journal of Psychiatric Research, 24*(4), 335–350.

Prien, R. F., Caffey, E. M., Klett, C. J. (1973). Prophylactic efficacy of lithium carbonate in manic-depressive illness. Report of the Veterans Administration and National Institute of Mental Health collaborative study group. *Archives of General Psychiatry, 28*(3), 337–341.

Quiroz, J. A., Yatham, L. N., Palumbo, J. M., Karcher, K., Kushner, S., & Kusumakar, V. (2010). Risperidone long-acting injectable monotherapy in the maintenance treatment of Bipolar I Disorder. *Biological Psychiatry, 68,* 56162, DOI: 10.1016/j.biopsych.2010.01.015

Rasgon, N. L., Reynolds, M. F., Elman, S., Frye, M., Bauer, M., & Altshuler, L. L. (2005). Longitudinal evaluation of reproductive function in women treated for bipolar disorder. *Journal of Affective Disorders, 89*(1–3), 217–225.

Rea, M. M., Tompson, M., Miklowitz, D. J., Goldstein, M. J., Hwang, S., & Mintz, J. (2003). Family focused treatment vs. individual treatment for Bipolar Disorder: Results of a randomized clinical trial. *Journal of Consulting and Clinical Psychology, 71*(3), 482–492.

Regier, D. A., Farmer, M. E., Rae, D. S., Locke, B. Z., Keith, S. J., Judd, L. L., et al. (1990). Comorbidity of mental disorders with alcohol and other drug abuse. Results from the Epidemiologic Catchment Area (ECA) Study. *Journal of the American Medical Association, 264*(19), 2511–2518.

Reilly-Harrington, N. A., Alloy, L. B., Fresco, D. M., & Whitehouse, W. G. (1999). Cognitive styles and life events interact to predict bipolar and unipolar symptomatology. *Journal of Abnormal Psychology, 108*(4), 567–578.

Robins, L. N., Marcus, L., Reich, W., Cunningham, R., & Gallagher, T. (1996). *Diagnostic Interview Schedule, Version IV.* St. Louis, MO: Department of Psychiatry, Washington School of Medicine.

Rogers, R. (1995). Diagnostic and structured interviewing: A handbook for psychologists. Odessa, FL: Psychological Assessment Resources.

Rush, A. J., Giles, D. E., Schlesser, M. A., Fulton, C. L., Weissenburger, J., & Burns, C. (1986). The Inventory for Depressive Symptomatology (IDS): Preliminary findings. *Psychiatry Research, 18*(1), 65–87.

Rush, A. J., Gullion, C. M., Basco, M. R., Jarrett, R. B., & Trivedi, M. H. (1996). The inventory of depressive symptomatology (IDS): Psychometric properties. *Psychological Medicine, 26,* 477–486.

Rush, A. J., Trivedi, M. H., Ibrahim, H. M., Carmody, T. J., Arnow, B., Klein, D. N., et al. (2003). The 16-item Quick Inventory of Depressive Symptomatology (QIDS) Clinician Rating (QIDS-C) and Self-Report (QIDS-SR): A psychometric evaluation in patients with chronic major depression. *Biological Psychiatry, 54,* 573–583.

Sachs, G., Chengappa, K. N., Suppes, T., Mullen, J. A., Brecher, M., Devine, N. A., et al. Quetiapine with lithium or divalproex for the treatment of bipolar mania: A randomized, double-blind, placebo-controlled study. *Bipolar Disord* 2004; 6:213–223.

Sachs, G., Sanchez, R., Marcus, R., Stock, E., McQuade, R., Carson, W., et al. (2006). Aripiprazole in the treatment of acute manic or mixed episodes in patients with bipolar I disorder: A 3-week placebo-controlled study. *Journal of Psychopharmacology, 20,* 536–546.

Sachs, G. S., Grossman, F., Ghaemi, S. N., Okamoto, A., & Bowden, C. L. Combination of a mood stabilizer with risperidone or haloperidol for treatment of acute mania: A double-blind, placebo-controlled comparison of efficacy and safety. *American Journal of Psychiatry, 159,* 1146–1154.

Sachs, G. S., Lafer, B., Stoll, A. L., Banov, M., Thibault, A. B., Tohen, M., et al. (1994). A double-blind trial of bupropion versus desipramine for bipolar depression. *Journal of Clinical Psychiatry, 55*(9), 391–393.

Sachs, G. S., Nierenberg, A. A., Calabrese, J. R., Marangell, L. B., Wisniewski, S. R., Gyulai, L., et al. (2007). Effectiveness of adjunctive antidepressant treatment for bipolar depression. *New England Journal of Medicine, 356,* 1711–1722.

Schaffer, A., Calrney, J., Cheung, A. H., Veldhuizen, S., & Levitt, A. J. (2006). Use of treatment services and pharmacotherapy for bipolar disorder in a general population-based mental health survey. *Journal of Clinical Psychiatry, 67,* 386–393.

Schneck, C. D., Miklowitz, D. J., Miyahara, S., Araga, M., Wisniewski, S., Gyulai, L., et al. (2008). The prospective course of rapid-cycling bipolar disorder: findings from the STEP-BD. *American Journal of Psychiatry, 165,* 370–377.

Scott, J., & Gutierrez, M. J. (2004). The current status of psychological treatments in bipolar disorders: A systematic review of relapse prevention. *Bipolar Disorders, 6*(6), 498–503.

Scott, J., Paykel, E., Morriss, R., Bentall, R., Kinderman, P., Johnson, T., et al. (2006). Cognitive behaviour therapy for severe and recurrent bipolar disorders: A randomised controlled trial. *British Journal of Psychiatry, 188,* 313–320.

Segal, J., Berk, M., & Brook, S. (1998). Risperidone compared with both lithium and haloperidol in mania: A double-blind randomized controlled trial. *Clinical Neuropharmacology, 21,* 176–180.

Simon, G. E., Ludman, E. J., Bauer, M. S., Unutzer, J., & Operskalski, B. Long-term effectiveness and cost of a systematic care program for bipolar disorder. *Archives of General Psychiatry, 63*(5), 500–508.

Simon, G. E., Ludman, E. J., Unutzer, J., Bauer, M. S., Operskalski, B., & Rutter, C. Randomized trial of a population-based care program for people with bipolar disorder. *Psychological Medicine, 35*(1), 13–24.

Small, J. G., Klapper, M. H., Kellams, J. J., Miller, M. J., Milstein, V., Sharpley, P. H., et al. (1988). Electroconvulsive treatment compared with lithium in the management of manic states. *Archives of General Psychiatry, 45*(8), 727–732.

Smoller, J. W., & Finn, C. T. (2003). Family, twin, and adoption studies of Bipolar Disorder. *American Journal of Medical Genetics, 123C,* 48–58.

Smulevich, A. B., Khanna, S., Eerdekens, M., Karcher, K., Kramer, M., & Grossman, F. (2005). Acute and continuation risperidone monotherapy in bipolar mania: A 3-week placebo-controlled trial followed by a 9-week double-blind trial of risperidone and haloperidol. *European Neuropsychopharmacology, 15*(1), 75–84.

Strakowski, S. M., DelBello, M. P., Fleck, D. E., & Arndt, S. (2000). The impact of substance abuse on the course of bipolar disorder. *Biological Psychiatry, 48*(6), 477–485.

Suppes, T., Anderson, R., Dennehy, D., Ozcan, M., Snow, D., & Sureddi, S. (2003). An open add-on study of oxcarbazepine versus divalproex to treat hypomanic symptoms in patients with Bipolar Disorder. Abstract presented at New Clinical Drug Evaluation Unit (NCDEU) 43rd Annual Meeting, Boca Raton, FL, May 27–30.

Suppes, T., Baldessarini, R. J., Faedda, G. L., & Tohen, M. (1991). Risk of recurrence following discontinuation of lithium treatment in Bipolar Disorder. *Archives of General Psychiatry, 48,* 1082–1088.

Suppes, T., Datto, C., Minkwitz, M., Nordenhem, A., Walker, C., Darko, D. Effectiveness of the extended release formulation of quetiapine as monotherapy for the treatment of acute bipolar depression. *Journal of Affective Disorders* 2010; 121: 106–115.

Suppes, T., & Dennehy, E. B. (2002). Evidence-based long-term treatment of bipolar II disorder. *Journal of Clinical Psychiatry, 63*(Suppl. 10), 29–33. Review.

Suppes, T., Dennehy, E. B., Hirschfeld, R. M. A., Altshuler, L. L., Bowden, C. L., Calabrese, J. R., et al. and the Texas Consensus Conference Panel on Medication Treatment of Bipolar Disorder. (2005). The Texas Implementation of Medication Algorithms: Update to the algorithms for treatment of bipolar I disorder. *Journal of Clinical Psychiatry. 66*(7), 870–886.

Suppes, T., Leverich, G. S., Keck, P. E., Nolen, W. A., Denicoff, K. D., Altshuler, L. L., et al. (2001). The Stanley Foundation Bipolar Treatment Outcome Network. II. Demographics and illness characteristics of the first 261 patients. *Journal of Affective Disorders, 67*(1–3), 45–59.

Suppes, T., Mintz, J., McElroy, S. L., Altshuler, L. L., Kupka, R. W., Frye, M. A., et al. (2005). Mixed hypomania in 908 patients with bipolar disorder evaluated prospectively in the Stanley Foundation Bipolar Treatment Network: A sex-specific phenomenon. *Archives of General Psychiatry, 62,* 1089–1096.

Suppes, T., Vieta, E., Liu, S., Brecher, M., & Paulsson, B. (2009). Maintenance treatment for patients with Bipolar I Disorder: Results from a North American study of quetiapine in combination with lithium or divalproex (Trial 127). *American Journal of Psychiatry, 166,* 476–488.

Suppes, T., Webb, A., Paul, B., Carmody, T., Kraemer, H., & Rush, A. J. (1999). Clinical outcome in a randomized 1-year trial of clozapine versus treatment as usual for patients with treatment-resistant illness and a history of mania. *American Journal of Psychiatry, 156*(8), 1164–1169.

Swann, A. C., Bowden, C. L., Morris, D., Calabrese, J. R., Petty, F., Small, J., et al. (1997). Depression during mania. Treatment response to lithium or divalproex. *Archives of General Psychiatry, 54*(1), 37–42.

Swartz, H. A., & Frank, E. (2001). Psychotherapy for bipolar depression: A phase specific treatment strategy? *Bipolar Disorders, 3,* 11–22.

Thase, M. E., Macfadden, W., Weisler, R. H., Chang, W., Paulsson, B., Khan, A., et al. (2006). Efficacy of quetiapine monotherapy in bipolar I and II depression: A double-blind, placebo-controlled study (the BOLDER II study). *Journal of Clinical Psychopharmacology, 26,* 600–609.

Thase, M. E., Mallinger, A. G., McKnight, D., & Himmelhoch, J. M. (1992). Treatment of imipramine-resistant recurrent depression, IV: A double-blind crossover study of tranylcypromine for anergic bipolar depression. *American Journal of Psychiatry, 149*(2), 195–198.

Tohen, M., Calabrese, J. R., Sachs, G. S., Banov, M. D., Detke, H. C., Risser, R., et al. (2006). Randomized, placebo-controlled trial of olanzapine as maintenance therapy in patients with bipolar I disorder responding to acute treatment with olanzapine. *American Journal of Psychiatry, 163,* 247–256.

Tohen, M., Chengappa, K. N. R., Suppes, T., Zarate, C. A., Calabrese, J. R., Bowden, C. L., et al. Efficacy of olanzapine in combination with valproate or lithium in the treatment of mania in patients partially nonresponsive to valproate or lithium monotherapy. *Arch Gen Psychiatry* 2002; 59:62–69.

Tohen, M., Greil, W., Calabrese, J. R., Sachs, G. S., Yatham, L. N., Oerlinghausen, B. M., et al. (2005). Olanzapine versus lithium in the maintenance treatment of bipolar disorder: A 12-month, randomized, double-blind, controlled clinical trial. *American Journal of Psychiatry, 162,* 1281–1290.

Tohen, M., Hennen, J., Zarate, C. M., Jr., Baldessarini, R. J., Strakowski, S. M., Stoll, A. L., et al. (2000). Two-year syndromal and functional recovery in 219 cases of first-episode major affective disorder with psychotic features. *American Journal of Psychiatry, 157*(2), 220–228.

Tohen, M., Jacobs, T. G., Grundy, S. L., McElroy, S. L., Banov, M. C., Janicak, P. G., et al. (2000). Efficacy of olanzapine in acute bipolar mania. *Archives of General Psychiatry, 57,* 841–849.

Tohen, M., Ketter, T. A., Zarate, C. A., Suppes, T., Frye, M., Altshuler, L., et al. (2003). Olanzapine versus divalproex sodium for the treatment of acute mania and maintenance of remission: A 47-week study. *American Journal of Psychiatry, 160,* 1263–1271.

Tohen, M., Sanger, T. M., McElroy, S. L., Tollefson, G. D., Chengappa, R., Daniel, D. G., et al. (1999). Olanzapine versus placebo in the treatment of acute mania. Olanzapine HGEH Study Group. *American Journal of Psychiatry, 156,* 702–709.

Tohen, M., Vieta, E., Calabrese, J., Ketter, T. A., Sachs, G., Bowden, C., et al. (2003). Efficacy of olanzapine and olanzapine-fluoxetine combination in the treatment of bipolar I depression. *Archives of General Psychiatry, 60,* 1079–1088.

Tohen, M., Waternaux, C. M., & Tsuang, M. T. (1990). Outcome in mania: A 4-year prospective follow-up of 75 patients utilizing survival analysis. *Archives of General Psychiatry, 47,* 1106–1111.

Tondo, L., Isacsson, G., & Baldessarini, R. J. (2003). Suicidal behaviour in bipolar disorder: Risk and prevention. *CNS Drugs, 17*(7), 491–511.

van der Loos, M. L., Mulder, P. G., Hartong, E. G., Blom, M. B., Vergouwen, A. C., de Keyzer, H. J. et al. (2009). Efficacy and safety of lamotrigine as add-on treatment to lithium in bipolar depression: A multicenter, double-blind, placebo-controlled trial. *Journal of Clinical Psychiatry, 70,* 223–231.

van Gent, E. M., & Zwart, F. M. (1991). Psychoeducation of partners of bipolar-manic patients. *Journal of Affective Disorders, 21*(1), 15–18.

Ventura, J., Nuechterlein, K. H., Subotnik, K., & Gilbert, E. (1995). Symptom dimension in recent-onset schizophrenia: The 24-item expanded BPRS. International Congress on Schizophrenia Research.

Vieta, E., Martinez-Aran, A., Goikolea, J. M., Torrent, C., Colom, F., Benabarre, A., et al. (2002). A randomized trial comparing paroxetine and venlafaxine in the treatment of bipolar depressed patients taking mood stabilizers. *Journal of Clinical Psychiatry, 63*(6), 508–512.

Vieta, E., Pacchiarotti, I., Valentí, M., Berk, L., Scott, J., & Colom, F. (2009). A critical update on psychological interventions for bipolar disorders. *Current Psychiatry Reports,* 11, 494–502.

Vieta, E., Suppes, T., Eggens, I., Persson, I., Paulsson, B., & Brecher, M. (2008b). Efficacy and safety of quetiapine in combination with lithium or divalproex for maintenance of patients with bipolar I disorder (international trial 126). *Journal of Affective Disorders, 109,* 251–263.

Wagner, K. D., Hirschfeld, R. M., Emslie, G. J., Findling, R. L., Gracious, B. L., & Reed, M. L. (2006). Validation of the Mood Disorder Questionnaire for bipolar disorders in adolescents. *Journal of Clinical Psychiatry, 67*(5), 827–830.

Wang, P. S., Berglund, P., Olfson, M., Pincus, H. A., Wells, K. B., & Kessler, R. C. (2005). Failure and delay in initial treatment contact after first onset of mental disorders in the National Comorbidity Survey Replication. *Archives of General Psychiatry, 62,* 603–613.

Weisler, R. H., Hirschfeld, R., Cutler, A. J., Gazda, T., Ketter, T. A., Keck, P. E. Jr., et al. (2006). Extended-release carbamazepine capsules as monotherapy in bipolar disorder: Pooled results from two randomised, double-blind, placebo-controlled trials. *CNS Drugs, 20*(3), 219–231.

Weisler, R. H., Kalali, A. H., & Ketter, T. A. (2004). A multicenter, randomized, double-blind, placebo-controlled trial of extended release carbamazepine capsules as monotherapy for bipolar disorder patients with manic or mixed episodes. *Journal of Clinical Psychiatry, 65,* 478–484.

Weissman, M. M., Markowitz, J., & Klerman, G. L. *Comprehensive guide to interpersonal psychotherapy.* New York: Basic Books.

Williams, J. B. W. (1988). A structured interview guide for the Hamilton Depression Rating Scale. *Archives of General Psychiatry, 45,* 742–747.

Yatham, L. N., Grossman, F., Augustyns, I., Vieta, E., & Ravindran, A. (2003). Mood stabilisers plus risperidone or placebo in the treatment of acute mania. International, double-blind, randomised controlled trial. *British Journal of Psychiatry, 182,* 141–147.

Yatham, L. N., Kennedy, S. H., Schaffer, A., Parikh, S. V., Beaulieu, S., O'Donovan, C., et al. (2009). Canadian Network for Mood and Anxiety Treatments (CANMAT) and International Society for Bipolar Disorders (ISBD) collaborative update of CANMAT guidelines for the management of patients with bipolar disorder: Update 2009. *Bipolar Disorders, 11,* 225–255.

Yatham, L. N., Paulsson, B., Mullen, J., & Vagero, A. M. Quetiapine versus placebo in combination with lithium or divalproex for the treatment of bipolar mania. *J Clin Psychopharmacol* 2004; 24: 599–606.

Young, A. H., McElroy, S. L., Bauer, M., Philips, N., Chang, W., Olausson, B., et al. A double-blind, placebo-controlled study of quetiapine and lithium monotherapy in adults in the acute phase of bipolar depression (Embolden I). *J Clinical Psychiatry* 2010; 71(2): 150–162.

Young, R. C., Biggs, J. T., Ziegler, B. E., & Mayer, D. A. (1978). A rating scale for mania: Reliability, validity and sensitivity. *British Journal of Psychiatry, 133,* 429–435.

Zarate, C. A., Jr., Payne, J. L., Singh, J., Quiroz, J. A., Luckenbaugh, D. A., Denicoff, K. D., et al. (2004). Pramipexole for bipolar II depression: A placebo-controlled proof of concept study. *Biological Psychiatry, 56,* 54–60.

Zaretsky, A., Lancee, W., Miller, C., Harris, A., Parikh, S. V. (2008). Is cognitive-behavioural therapy more effective than psychoeducation in bipolar disorder? *Canadian Journal of Psychiatry, 53*(7), 441–448.

Zaretsky, A. E., Rizvi, S., & Parikh, S. V. (2007). How well do psychosocial interventions work in bipolar disorder? *Canadian Journal of Psychiatry, 52*(1), 14–21.

Zimmermann, P., Brückl, T., Nocon, A., Pfister, H., Lieb, R., Wittchen, H., et al. Heterogeneity of DSM-IV major depressive disorder as a consequence of subthreshold bipolarity. *Archives of General Psychiatry, 66,* 1341–1352.

Index

Note: Italicized page locators indicate a figure; tables are noted with a *t*.

A

Absolute starting dose, 42
Activating events, 67
Active listening, 64–65
ADHD (attention deficit/hyperactivity disorder), 28
Affect, defined, 21
Alcohol abuse, 9, 53
Algorithms, defined, 32
AMRS (Altman Mania Rating Scale), 92
Amygdala, 5
Anticonvulsant medications
    and depression, 47
    dosages and side effects, *35*
    in maintenance treatment, 49–50
    trade names of, *34*
Antidepressants
    dosages and side effects, 43*t*
    in maintenance treatment, 50–51
    and mania/hypomania, 44–45
    trade names of, *34*
Antipsychotics, second-generation
    and depression, 42, 44,
      46–47
    dosages and side effects, *36*, 44*t*
    in maintenance treatment, 50
    and mania/hypomania, 37–38
    monitoring protocol for, 41*t*
    trade names for, *34*
Anxiety disorders, 28–29, 54
Aripiprazole
    dosages and side effects, 36*t*
    FDA indications for, 33*t*
    in maintenance treatment, 48–49, 50
    and mania/hypomania, 37, 39
    trade names, 34*t*
Asenapine
    dosages and side effects, 36*t*
    FDA indications for trade names, 33*t*
    and mania/hypomania, 37, 39
    trade names, 34*t*
Attention deficit hyperactivity disorder (ADHD), 28
Attributional styles, 57
Atypical features, defined, 17, 19

B

Beck Depression Inventory (BDI-2), 93
Beck Hopelessness Scale (BHS), 26
Beck Scale for Suicide Ideation (BSS), 25
Behavioral rehearsal, 65
Beliefs, defined, 67
Bipolar diagnostic criteria, *18,* 77–86
Bipolar disorder
    causes of, 2
    course specifiers for, 19
    defined, 2
    diagnosis of, 87–88
    not otherwise specified (BD NOS),
      defined, 17
    and other disorders, 26–29
    physiological causes of, 20–21
    prevalence of, 11
    tools for diagnosis of, 19–26
Bipolar I Disorder (BDI), 17, 32, 80–84
Bipolar II Disorder (BDII), 17, 32, 84–86
Brain, involvement of, 5–6, *6,* 11
Brief Psychiatric Rating Scale (BPRS), 93–94
Bupropion, 45

C

Carbamazepine
    dosages and side effects, 35*t*
    FDA indications for, 33*t*
    in maintenance treatment, 50
    and mania/hypomania, 37, 39
    trade names, 34*t*
CARS-M (Clinician Administered Rating Scale for Mania), 90
Catatonic features, defined, 17
CBT (cognitive behavioral therapy), 67–70, 73–74
CCM (chronic care management), 63–64, 73–74
Change, coping with, 71–72
Children/adolescents, 16, 29, 33
Circadian rhythms, 8, 72. *See also* Insomnia
Clinician Administered Rating Scale for Mania (CARS-M), 90
Clozapine
    dosages and side effects, 36*t,* 52
    in maintenance, 50
    and mania/hypomania, 37, 39–40
    trade names for, 34*t*

Co-occuring disorders, 53–54
Cognitive behavioral therapy (CBT), 67–70
    compared with other therapies, 73–74
Communication, assertive, 65
Communication enhancement training, 64–65
Conflicts, interpersonal, 71
Consequences, defined, 67
Crossover design, defined, 38
Cyclothymic disorder, defined, 17

D

DBSA (Depression and Bipolar Support
    Alliance), 92, 96
Delusions, defined, 15
Depression
    and bipolar disorder, 13, 42–47, 43*t*
    in children/adolescents, 29
    defined, 2
    effectiveness of medications, 45–47
    impact of, 9–10
    misdiagnosis of, 32
    and OFC, 46
    rating scales for, 23
    symptoms of, *14,* 16, 96
Depressive episodes, 16, 17, *18,*
    77–78
Depressive symptoms, 47, 70
Derailment, 19
Diabetes, and second-generation
    antipsychotics, 40–41
*Diagnostic and Statistical Manual of Mental
    Disorders* (APA), 2
Diagnostic criteria, dimensions of, 3–4
Diagnostic Interview Schedule (DIS),
    87–88
Diagnostic specifiers, bipolar I disorder and
    bipolar II disorder, 17–19
Dopamine, 7
Drug interactions, 51
DSM–IV–TR, criteria for bipolar disorder, 17
Dysphoria, defined, 13

E

Electroconvulsive therapy (ECT), 51, 53
Emergent episodes, warning signs of, 58
Epilepsy, 20, 27–28, 53
Episodes, time between, 3
Euthymia, defined, 2
Executive functions, defined, 5

F

Family-Focused Treatment (FFT), 64–67,
    73–74
Feelings, expression of, 65

G

Genetics, role of, 4–5
Goals, for CBT patients, 68–69
Grandiosity, 8, 78, 79
Grief, 70–71

H

Hallucinations, defined, 15
Hamilton Rating Scale for Depression
    (HAM-D), 90–91
Head injuries, 21, 27–28
Hippocampus, 5
Hopelessness, 26
Hyperandrogenism, 38
Hypomania
    in assessments, 13
    defined, 2, 15
    impact of, 9
    mixed, 10
    symptoms of, *14,* 15, 96
Hypomanic episodes, *18,* 79–80

I

IDS-C (Inventory of Depressive
    Symptomatology-Clinician Rated), 91
IDS-SR, 92–93
Impairment, functional, 58–59
Impulsivity, defined, 2
Insight, defined, 24
Insomnia, 8, 52*t,* 77. *See also* Circadian
    rhythms
Intensive clinical management (ICM), 72–73
Interpersonal skill deficits, 72
Interpersonal Social Rhythm Therapy (IPSRT),
    70–74
Interrater reliability, defined, 90
Interviews
    checklist for, *22*
    conducting of, 21
    self-adminstered, 87–88
    structured, 21–23
    Inventory of Depressive Symptomatology–
        Clinician Rated (IDS-C), 91
    IPSRT (Interpersonal Social Rhythm
        Therapy), 70–74
    ISS, 92

L

Lamotrigine, 46, 49
Life Chart, 62, 92, 95–99
Life Goals Program, 63
Lithium
    and depression, 42, 45

dosages and side effects, *35,* 43*t*
FDA indications for, 33*t*
in maintenance treatment, 49
and mania/hypomania, 38
trade names for, *34*

M

MADRS (Montgomery-Äsberg Depression
    Rating Scale), 91
Maintenance treatment, 37, 48–51, 69–70
Major depressive disorder (MDD), 27
Mania
    in children/adolescents, 29
    imaging of, *6*
    symptoms of, *14,* 14–15, 96
Manic episodes
    characteristics of, *18*
    criteria for, 78–79
    defined, 15
    effect of, 8
    specifiers for, 17, 19
MAOIs (monoamine oxidase inhibitors), *34*
MCMI-III (Millon Clinical Multiaxial
    Inventory), 93, 94
MDD (major depressive disorder), 27
MDQ (Mood Disorders Questionnaire), 24,
    88–89
Medical conditions, and mood disorders, 27–28
Medication therapy
    adherence to, 56, 61, 62
    and FFT, 66
Medications. *See also specific drugs*
    balance of, 26
    discontinuation of, 11, 56
    dosages and side effects, 35–36, 43*t*
    FDA indications, 33*t*
    tapering of, 48
    trade names for, *34*
    used for depression, 42–47
    used for maintenance, 48–51
    used for mania/hypomania, 33–41
    using combination, 41
Melancholic features, defined, 17
Messenger systems, secondary, 7–8
Millon Clinical Multiaxial Inventory
    (MCMI-III), 93, 94
Minnesota Multiphasic Personality
    Inventory–2nd Edition (MMPI-2), 93, 94
Mixed episodes
    in assessments, 13
    characteristics of, *18*
    criteria for, 79
    defined, 13

impact of, 10
    recognizing, 16
Monoamine oxidase inhibitors (MAOIs), *34*
Montgomery-Äsberg Depression Rating Scale
    (MADRS), 91
Mood disorder, substance-induced, 27
Mood Disorders Questionnaire (MDQ), 24,
    88–89
Moods, tracking of, 97

N

Neoplastic/cancer syndromes, 20, 27–28
Neurochemical receptor groups, major, 7
Neuroprotective effect, 7
Neurotransmitters, 7

O

Obesity, and second-generation antipsychotics,
    40–41
Olanzapine
    and depression, 45
    dosages and side effects, 36*t*
    FDA indications for, 33*t*
    and mania/hypomania, 40
    trade names, 34*t*
Olanzapine-fluoxetine combination (OFC), 47
    and depression, 42, 44, 47
    dosages and side effects, 44*t*
    FDA indications for, 33*t*
    trade names, 34*t*

P

Paranormal phenomena, 6
Patient history, taking, 4
Patients' lives, effect on, 8–10
Patterns, individual, 2–3, *6*
PET imaging, 2, 6
Physicians' Desk Reference, 35, 51
Polycystic ovarian syndrome, 38
Pramipexole
    and depression, 42
    dosages and side effects, 43*t,* 46
    trade name, 34*t*
Problem-solving, 60*t,* 65
Psychoeducation
    defined, 61
    effectiveness of, 63–64
    for families, 64
    use of, 56, 59, 60*t*
Psychotherapy, in maintenance, 58
Psychotic disorders, 28

Q

Quality of life, 58–59
Quetiapine
      and depression, 42, 46–47
      dosages and side effects, 36t, 44t
      FDA indications for, 33t
      and mania/hypomania, 37, 40
      trade names, 34t
Quick Inventory of Depressive
      Symptomatology–Clinician Rated
      (QIDS-C), 91

R

Rapid cycling, 13, 19
Rating scales, observational, *22, 23*
Recovery, likelihood of, 11
Relapses, 58, 61–62
Repetitive transcranial magnetic stimulation
      (rTMS), 53
Research, brain, 7–8
Risperidone
      dosages and side effects, 36t
      FDA indications for, 33t
      and mania/hypomania, 37, 40
      trade names, 34t
Role-playing, 65
Role transitions, 71–72
rTMS (repetitive transcranial magnetic
      stimulation), 53

S

Scale for Suicide Ideation (SSI), 25–26
Schedule for Affective Disorders and
      Schizophrenia (SADS), 87
SCID (Structured Clinical Interview), 88, 89
Screening instruments, self-administered,
      88–89
Seasonal pattern, defined, 19
Self-ratings, 23–24
Self-report tools, 24
Sensitivity, defined, 89
Serotonin, 7
Side effects, management of, 51, 52t
SIS (Suicide Intent Scale), 26
Sleep-wake cycles, 57. *See also* Circadian
      rhythms
Social support, importance of, 57
Somatization, 87
Specificity, defined, 89
Specifiers, defined, 17
SPECT imaging, 6, *6*
SSI (Scale for Suicide Ideation), 25–26
SSRI medications, 43t, 45, 47
Stevens Johnson syndrome, 46

Stress
      coping with, 57
      effect of, 3, 5
      and IPSRT, 72
      managing, 62
Strokes, embolic, 20, 27–28
Structured Clinical Interview (SCID), 88, 89
Substance abuse. *See also* Alcohol abuse
      impact of, 9, 78
      and medical treatment, 53–54
      and mood disorders, 27–28
      prevalence of, 9
      risk for, 5
Suicide Intent Scale (SIS), 26
Suicide risk, 10, 25–26, 77
Symptoms
      assessment of, 89–91
      self-rating of, 91–93
      typical, 13–16

T

T-scores, 94
Tangentiality, 19
Temporal lobe, 5
Thyroid conditions, 20, 27–28
Titration, rate of initial, 42
Trazadone, 45
Twins, and risk of bipolar disorder, 4

V

Vagal nerve stimulation, 53
Valproate
      and depression, 42, 46
      dosages and side effects, 35t, 43t
      FDA indications for, 33t
      in maintenance treatment, 49–50
      and mania/hypomania, 37, 38, 42
      trade names, 34t
Venlafaxine, 45

W

Wellness, 58

Y

Young Mania Rating Scale (YMRS), 89–90

Z

Ziprasidone
      dosages and side effects, 36t
      FDA indications for, 33t
      and mania/hypomania, 40
      trade name, 34t